This report contains the collective views of an international group of experts and does not necessarily represent the decisions or the stated policy of the World Health Organization, the International Labour Organization, or the United Nations Environment Programme.

Harmonization Project Document No. 4

PART 1: IPCS FRAMEWORK FOR ANALYSING THE RELEVANCE OF A CANCER MODE OF ACTION FOR HUMANS AND CASE-STUDIES

PART 2: IPCS FRAMEWORK FOR ANALYSING THE RELEVANCE OF A NON-CANCER MODE OF ACTION FOR HUMANS

This project was conducted within the IPCS project on the Harmonization of Approaches to the Assessment of Risk from Exposure to Chemicals.

Published under the joint sponsorship of the World Health Organization, the International Labour Organization, and the United Nations Environment Programme, and produced within the framework of the Inter-Organization Programme for the Sound Management of Chemicals.

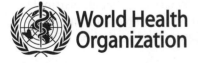

The **International Programme on Chemical Safety (IPCS)**, established in 1980, is a joint venture of the United Nations Environment Programme (UNEP), the International Labour Organization (ILO), and the World Health Organization (WHO). The overall objectives of the IPCS are to establish the scientific basis for assessment of the risk to human health and the environment from exposure to chemicals, through international peer review processes, as a prerequisite for the promotion of chemical safety, and to provide technical assistance in strengthening national capacities for the sound management of chemicals.

The **Inter-Organization Programme for the Sound Management of Chemicals (IOMC)** was established in 1995 by UNEP, ILO, the Food and Agriculture Organization of the United Nations, WHO, the United Nations Industrial Development Organization, the United Nations Institute for Training and Research, and the Organisation for Economic Co-operation and Development (Participating Organizations), following recommendations made by the 1992 UN Conference on Environment and Development to strengthen cooperation and increase coordination in the field of chemical safety. The purpose of the IOMC is to promote coordination of the policies and activities pursued by the Participating Organizations, jointly or separately, to achieve the sound management of chemicals in relation to human health and the environment.

WHO Library Cataloguing-in-Publication Data

IPCS mode of action framework.

(IPCS harmonization project document ; no. 4)

1.Hazardous substances – toxicity. 2.Risk assessment – methods. 3.Risk management – methods. 4.Carcinogenicity tests. 5.Carcinogens. 6. Neoplasms – chemically induced. I.International Programme on Chemical Safety. II.Series.

ISBN 978 92 4 156349 9   (NLM classification: QV 602)

TABLE OF CONTENTS

FOREWORD

Harmonization Project Documents are a family of publications by the World Health Organization (WHO) under the umbrella of the International Programme on Chemical Safety (IPCS) (WHO/ILO/UNEP). Harmonization Project Documents complement the Environmental Health Criteria (EHC) methodology (yellow cover) series of documents as authoritative documents on methods for the risk assessment of chemicals.

The main impetus for the current coordinated international, regional, and national efforts on the assessment and management of hazardous chemicals arose from the 1992 United Nations Conference on Environment and Development (UNCED). UNCED Agenda 21, Chapter 19, provides the "blueprint" for the environmentally sound management of toxic chemicals. This commitment by governments was reconfirmed at the 2002 World Summit on Sustainable Development and in 2006 in the Strategic Approach to International Chemicals Management (SAICM). The IPCS project on the Harmonization of Approaches to the Assessment of Risk from Exposure to Chemicals (Harmonization Project) is conducted under Agenda 21, Chapter 19, and contributes to the implementation of SAICM. In particular, the project addresses the SAICM objective on Risk Reduction and the SAICM Global Plan of Action activity to "Develop and use new and harmonized methods for risk assessment".

The IPCS Harmonization Project goal is *to improve chemical risk assessment globally, through the pursuit of common principles and approaches, and, hence, strengthen national and international management practices that deliver better protection of human health and the environment within the framework of sustainability.* The Harmonization Project aims to harmonize global approaches to chemical risk assessment, including by developing international guidance documents on specific issues. The guidance is intended for adoption and use in countries and by international bodies in the performance of chemical risk assessments. The guidance is developed by engaging experts worldwide. The project has been implemented using a stepwise approach, first sharing information and increasing understanding of methods and practices used by various countries, identifying areas where convergence of different approaches would be beneficial, and then developing guidance that enables implementation of harmonized approaches. The project uses a building block approach, focusing at any one time on the aspects of risk assessment that are particularly important for harmonization.

The project enables risk assessments (or components thereof) to be performed using internationally accepted methods, and these assessments can then be shared to avoid duplication and optimize use of valuable resources for risk management. It also promotes sound science as a basis for risk management decisions, promotes transparency in risk assessment, and reduces unnecessary testing of chemicals. Advances in scientific knowledge can be translated into new harmonized methods.

This ongoing project is overseen by a geographically representative Harmonization Project Steering Committee and a number of ad hoc Working Groups that manage the detailed work. Finalization of documents includes a rigorous process of international peer review and public comment.

1

IPCS FRAMEWORK FOR ANALYSING THE RELEVANCE OF A CANCER MODE OF ACTION FOR HUMANS AND CASE-STUDIES

PREFACE

Following publication of the International Programme on Chemical Safety (IPCS) Conceptual Framework for Evaluating a Mode of Action for Chemical Carcinogenesis (in animals),[1] an IPCS Cancer Working Group convened on 3–5 March 2004 in Arlington, Virginia, USA. The working group agreed that the issue of human relevance of animal tumours should be further explored with the goal of developing a unified IPCS Human Relevance Framework for use of mode of action information in risk assessment for regulatory and other purposes, and it provided initial guidance for this task. The members of this working group, including secretariat support and a representative of the Organisation for Economic Co-operation and Development, were as follows:

Professor Hermann Bolt, Institut für Arbeitsphysiologie, Germany
Professor Alan R. Boobis, Department of Health Toxicology Unit, Imperial College London, United Kingdom
Dr John Bucher, National Institute of Environmental Health Sciences, USA
Dr Vincent Cogliano, Unit of Carcinogen Identification and Evaluation, International Agency for Research on Cancer, France
Dr Samuel M. Cohen, Pathology and Microbiology, Havlik-Wall Professor of Oncology, University of Nebraska Medical Center, USA
Dr William Farland, Office of Research and Development, Environmental Protection Agency, USA
Dr Jun Kanno, Division of Cellular & Molecular Toxicology, National Institute of Health Sciences, Japan
Dr Lois D. Lehman-McKeeman, Bristol-Myers Squibb, USA
Ms Bette Meek, Environmental Health Centre, Health Canada, Canada
Ms Laurence Musset, Environment, Health and Safety Division, Organisation for Economic Co-operation and Development, France
Dr Jerry Rice, Consultant, USA
Ms Cindy Sonich-Mullin, International Programme on Chemical Safety, World Health Organization, USA
Ms Carolyn Vickers, International Programme on Chemical Safety, World Health Organization, Switzerland
Ms Deborah Willcocks, Existing Chemicals, National Industrial Chemicals Notification and Assessment Scheme (NICNAS), Australia

Extending the Mode of Action Framework to include consideration of human relevance, taking into account guidance from the Arlington meeting, was the subject of an IPCS international workshop convened in Bradford, United Kingdom, from 21 to 23 April 2005. This workshop prepared draft text for an IPCS Human Relevance Framework, including updating the 2001 Mode of Action Framework. The workshop participants, including

---

[1] Sonich-Mullin C, Fielder R, Wiltse J, Baetcke K, Dempsey J, Fenner-Crisp P, Grant D, Hartley M, Knaap A, Kroese D, Mangelsdorf I, Meek E, Rice J, Younes M (2001) IPCS conceptual framework for evaluating a mode of action for chemical carcinogenesis. *Regulatory Toxicology and Pharmacology*, **34**:146–152.

secretariat support and representatives of the European Food Safety Authority and European Chemicals Bureau, were as follows:

Dr Peter Abbott, Scientific Risk Assessment and Evaluation Branch, Food Standards Australia New Zealand, Australia

Dr Antero Aitio, International Programme on Chemical Safety, World Health Organization, Switzerland

Dr Diana Anderson, Department of Biomedical Sciences, University of Bradford, United Kingdom

Professor Sir Colin Berry, United Kingdom

Professor Hermann Bolt, Institut für Arbeitsphysiologie, Germany

Professor Alan R. Boobis, Department of Health Toxicology Unit, Imperial College London, United Kingdom

Dr Susy Brescia, Health and Safety Executive, United Kingdom

Dr John Bucher, National Institute of Environmental Health Sciences, USA

Dr Vincent Cogliano, Unit of Carcinogen Identification and Evaluation, International Agency for Research on Cancer, France

Dr Samuel M. Cohen, Pathology and Microbiology, Havlik-Wall Professor of Oncology, University of Nebraska Medical Center, USA

Dr Vicki Dellarco, Office of Pesticide Programs, Environmental Protection Agency, USA

Ms Christine Dove, School of Life Sciences, University of Bradford, United Kingdom

Dr Jun Kanno, Division of Cellular and Molecular Toxicology, National Institute of Health Sciences, Japan

Dr Janet Kielhorn, Department of Chemical Risk Assessment, Fraunhofer Institute for Toxicology and Experimental Medicine, Germany

Mrs Sandra Kunz, International Programme on Chemical Safety, World Health Organization, Switzerland

Dr Christian Laurent, Scientific Expert Services, European Food Safety Authority, Italy

Dr Douglas McGregor, Toxicity Evaluation Consultants, United Kingdom

Ms Bette Meek, Environmental Health Centre, Health Canada, Canada

Ms Sharon Munn, Toxicology and Chemical Substances, European Chemicals Bureau, Italy

Dr R. Julian Preston, National Health and Environmental Effects Research Laboratory, Environmental Carcinogenesis Division, Environmental Protection Agency, USA

Dr Jerry Rice, Consultant, USA

Dr Hans-Bernhard Richter-Reichhelm, Federal Institute for Risk Assessment (BfR), Germany

Ms Carolyn Vickers, International Programme on Chemical Safety, World Health Organization, Switzerland

Ms Deborah Willcocks, Existing Chemicals, National Industrial Chemicals Notification and Assessment Scheme (NICNAS), Australia

Dr William P. Wood, Risk Assessment Forum, Environmental Protection Agency, USA

Dr Zheng Yuxin, Institute for Occupational Health and Poison Control, Chinese Center for Disease Control and Prevention, and WHO Collaborating Centre of Occupational Health, People's Republic of China

The draft was published on the Internet for public comment and sent to a number of WHO Collaborating Centres and IPCS Participating Institutions for peer review. An expert meeting that convened in London in December 2005 considered the comments received and finalized the framework. The expert meeting participants were as follows:

Professor Alan R. Boobis, Department of Health Toxicology Unit, Imperial College London, United Kingdom *(Rapporteur)*

Dr Samuel M. Cohen, Pathology and Microbiology, Havlik-Wall Professor of Oncology, University of Nebraska Medical Center, USA

Dr Vicki Dellarco, Office of Pesticide Programs, Environmental Protection Agency, USA

Dr William Farland, Office of Research and Development, Environmental Protection Agency, USA *(Chair)*

Dr Douglas McGregor, Toxicity Evaluation Consultants, United Kingdom

Ms Carolyn Vickers, International Programme on Chemical Safety, World Health Organization, Switzerland

Ms Deborah Willcocks, Existing Chemicals, National Industrial Chemicals Notification and Assessment Scheme (NICNAS), Australia

LIST OF CONTRIBUTORS

Sir Colin Berry
Emeritus Professor of Biology, Queen Mary, London, United Kingdom

Hermann Bolt
Institut für Arbeitsphysiologie, Dortmund, Germany

Alan R. Boobis
Experimental Medicine and Toxicology, Division of Medicine, Imperial College London, London, United Kingdom

Vincent Cogliano
Carcinogen Identification and Evaluation Unit, International Agency for Research on Cancer, Lyon, France

Samuel M. Cohen
Department of Pathology and Microbiology and Eppley Institute for Cancer Research, University of Nebraska Medical Center, Omaha, Nebraska, USA

Vicki Dellarco
Office of Pesticide Programs, Environmental Protection Agency, Washington, DC, USA

William Farland
Office of Research and Development, Environmental Protection Agency, Washington, DC, USA

Douglas McGregor
Toxicity Evaluation Consultants, Aberdour, United Kingdom

M.E. (Bette) Meek
Existing Substances Division, Safe Environments Programme, Health Canada, Ottawa, Ontario, Canada

R. Julian Preston
Environmental Protection Agency, Research Triangle Park, North Carolina, USA

Hans-Bernhard Richter-Reichhelm
Federal Institute for Risk Assessment (BfR), Berlin, Germany

Carolyn Vickers
International Programme on Chemical Safety, World Health Organization, Geneva, Switzerland

Deborah Willcocks
National Industrial Chemicals Notification and Assessment Scheme, Sydney, Australia

LIST OF ACRONYMS AND ABBREVIATIONS

ADH	alcohol dehydrogenase
ANOVA	analysis of variance
bw	body weight
CAR	constitutively active receptor
cDNA	complementary deoxyribonucleic acid
CoA	coenzyme A
CpG	cytosine and guanine separated by a phosphate
CYP	cytochrome P-450
dA	deoxyadenosine
dG	deoxyguanosine
DMSO	dimethyl sulfoxide
DNA	deoxyribonucleic acid
DPX	DNA–protein cross-links
FAO	Food and Agriculture Organization of the United Nations
HRF	Human Relevance Framework
IARC	International Agency for Research on Cancer
ILO	International Labour Organization
ILSI	International Life Sciences Institute
IPCS	International Programme on Chemical Safety
IU	International Units
JMPR	Joint FAO/WHO Meeting on Pesticide Residues
K_M	Michaelis-Menten constant
LOAEL	lowest-observed-adverse-effect level
MOA	mode of action
NAT	*N*-acetyltransferase
NOAEL	no-observed-adverse-effect level
NTP	National Toxicology Program (USA)
OAT	*O*-acetyltransferase
PCNA	proliferating cell nuclear antigen
PPX	protein–protein cross-linkage
RNA	ribonucleic acid
RSI	Risk Science Institute (ILSI)
rT3	reverse triiodothyronine
S9	$9000 \times g$ supernatant from rat liver
SCE	sister chromatid exchange
SHE	Syrian hamster embryo
T3	triiodothyronine
T4	thyroxine
TCDD	2,3,7,8-tetrachlorodibenzo-*p*-dioxin
TGF	tumour growth factor
TSH	thyroid stimulating hormone
UDP	uridine diphosphate
UDS	unscheduled DNA synthesis
UGT	uridine diphosphate glucuronosyltransferase

ULLI	unit length labelling index
UNEP	United Nations Environment Programme
USA	United States of America
USEPA	United States Environmental Protection Agency
WHO	World Health Organization

IPCS FRAMEWORK FOR ANALYSING THE RELEVANCE OF A CANCER MODE OF ACTION FOR HUMANS[1]

Alan R. Boobis, Samuel M. Cohen, Vicki Dellarco, Douglas McGregor,
M.E. (Bette) Meek, Carolyn Vickers, Deborah Willcocks, & William Farland

The use of structured frameworks can be invaluable in promoting harmonization in the assessment of chemical risk. The International Programme on Chemical Safety (IPCS) has therefore updated and extended its Mode of Action (MOA) Framework for cancer to address the issue of human relevance of a carcinogenic response observed in an experimental study. The first stage is to determine whether it is possible to establish an MOA. This comprises a series of key events along the causal pathway to cancer, identified using a weight-of-evidence approach based on the Bradford Hill criteria. The key events are then compared first qualitatively and then quantitatively between the experimental animals and humans. Finally, a clear statement of confidence, analysis, and implications is produced. The IPCS Human Relevance Framework for cancer provides an analytical tool to enable the transparent evaluation of the data, identification of key data gaps, and structured presentation of information that would be of value in the further risk assessment of the compound, even if relevancy cannot be excluded. This might include data on the shape of the dose–response curve, identification of any thresholds, and recognition of potentially susceptible subgroups, for example, the basis of genetic or life stage differences.

Fundamental to the evolution of cancer risk assessment over the last three decades has been our increasing understanding of the biology of cancer and the identification of key events in carcinogenesis. Through the mid-1980s, national and international assessments of human cancer hazard and risk depended primarily on lifetime assays in rodents of potentially carcinogenic agents. For few agents was there sufficient human evidence on which to base retrospective cancer assessments, and fewer still would be expected to be detected prospectively, given modern controls on general exposures in the workplace and in the environment generally. Inherent in rodent-based assessments was the assumption that the observation of tumours in laboratory animals could be meaningfully extrapolated to identify potential human carcinogens and, by the use of mathematical models, to provide upper-bound estimates of risk at human doses of regulatory significance. During the same period, the potential significance of mutagenesis in carcinogenesis was becoming accepted by the scientific community. Subsequently, it has become increasingly apparent that an appreciable number of chemicals cause cancer in laboratory animals by processes that do not involve direct interaction with DNA. These developments in our understanding of the biological basis of carcinogenesis in both laboratory animals and humans have benefited risk assessment processes by providing more data on the pharmacokinetics and pharmacodynamics of suspect carcinogenic agents. Consideration of the biological processes involved in the carcinogenesis of specific compounds has led to the concept of mode of action (MOA).

---

[1] This article, to which WHO owns copyright, was originally published in 2006 in *Critical Reviews in Toxicology*, Volume 36, pages 781–792. It has been edited for this WHO publication and includes corrigenda.

A postulated MOA for carcinogenesis is a biologically plausible sequence of key events leading to an observed effect supported by robust experimental observations and mechanistic data. It describes key cytological and biochemical events—that is, those that are both measurable and necessary to the observed carcinogenicity—in a logical framework. MOA contrasts with mechanism of action, which generally involves a sufficient understanding of the molecular basis for an effect and its detailed description so that causation can be established in molecular terms.

In 2001, as part of its efforts to harmonize risk assessment practices, the International Programme on Chemical Safety (IPCS) (WHO/ILO/UNEP) published a framework for assessment of MOA for carcinogenesis in laboratory animals (animal MOA), based on Bradford Hill criteria for causality. The IPCS Human Relevance Framework (HRF) presented in this document updates this MOA Framework and extends it to consider human relevance. It is an analytical tool to provide a means of evaluating systematically the data available on a specific carcinogenic response to a chemical in a transparent manner. While it is envisaged that the framework will be of value to risk assessors both within and outside of regulatory agencies, it will also be a valuable tool to the research community. Among reasons for using the framework are:

- to provide a generic approach to the analysis of data to contribute to harmonization;
- to encourage transparency of the consideration and use of available data and reasons for the conclusions drawn;
- to provide guidance in the presentation of data;
- to identify critical data deficiencies and needs;
- to inform the quantitative assessment of carcinogenic risk to humans.

These and other topics will be discussed in more detail below.

THE ROLE OF IPCS IN DEVELOPING THE FRAMEWORK FOR ANALYSING THE RELEVANCE OF A CANCER MOA FOR HUMANS

IPCS has been leading an effort to harmonize approaches to cancer risk assessment as part of its larger project on the Harmonization of Approaches to the Assessment of Risk from Exposure to Chemicals. The first phase of this work resulted in the publication of the IPCS Conceptual Framework for Evaluating a Mode of Action for Chemical Carcinogenesis in experimental animals (Sonich-Mullin et al., 2001). As described in that publication, a major impediment to harmonization identified in the consideration of weight of evidence was the evaluation of MOA in animals. Sonich-Mullin et al. (2001) provided a framework for evaluating MOA of chemical carcinogenesis in animals and recognized the importance of moving on to the next step in the overall characterization of cancer hazard and risk in humans: the assessment of relevance of the MOA of animal carcinogenesis to humans. Adoption of the MOA Framework concept is proceeding through its incorporation in the revised United States Environmental Protection Agency (USEPA) Guidelines for Carcinogen Risk Assessment (USEPA, 1999, 2005), and the framework is now commonly used by other regulatory agencies and international organizations. In the United Kingdom, the framework is being used for the assessment of pesticides and industrial chemicals. The United Kingdom

Committee on Carcinogenicity (2004) has noted the framework's value with regard to both harmonization between agencies and internal consistency in its latest guidelines. The framework has also been adopted and is being used by agencies in Australia and in Canada, in the evaluation of Existing Chemicals under the Canadian Environmental Protection Act. The European Union has incorporated the framework into its technical guidance documents on evaluating new and existing industrial chemicals and biocides, including carcinogenicity. With regard to international organizations, of particular note is the use of the framework by the Joint FAO/WHO Meeting on Pesticide Residues (JMPR), for example, in its evaluation of pyrethrin extract and its incorporation into the resulting monograph.

The step to extend the MOA Framework to include consideration of human relevance has been undertaken by IPCS in cooperation with international partners. It was the subject of an IPCS international workshop convened in Bradford, United Kingdom, from 21 to 23 April 2005. This workshop prepared draft text for an IPCS HRF, including updating the 2001 MOA Framework. The draft was published on the Internet for public comment and sent to a number of WHO Collaborating Centres and IPCS Participating Institutions for peer review. An expert meeting convened in London in December 2005 considered the comments received and finalized the framework. The framework text and the steps leading to its development are discussed in detail in the following sections.

THE 2001 IPCS CONCEPTUAL MOA FRAMEWORK FOR EVALUATING ANIMAL CARCINOGENESIS

Purpose of the framework

The IPCS MOA Framework for evaluating carcinogenesis in animals (Sonich-Mullin et al., 2001) remains a fundamental basis for the IPCS Framework for Analysing the Relevance of a Cancer Mode of Action for Humans. The animal MOA Framework provides a generic approach to the principles commonly used when evaluating a postulated MOA for tumour induction in animals by a chemical carcinogen. Thus, the framework is a tool that provides a structured approach to the assessment of the overall weight of the evidence for the postulated MOA. In this context, a supported MOA would have evidence provided by robust experimental observations and mechanistic data to establish a biologically plausible explanation.

The framework is designed to bring transparency to the analysis of a postulated MOA and thereby promote confidence in the conclusions reached through the use of a defined procedure that encourages clear and consistent documentation supporting the analysis and reasoning and that highlights inconsistencies and uncertainties in the available data. The purpose of the framework is to provide a systematic means of considering the weight of the evidence for an MOA in a given situation; it is not designed to give an absolute answer on sufficiency of the information, as this will vary depending on the circumstance. It is not a checklist of criteria, but rather an analytical approach. However, the process can be greatly aided by the presentation of tabular summaries of comparative data on incidence of key events and tumours.

The animal MOA Framework analysis is an important step in the hazard characterization. It is envisaged that the animal MOA Framework will contribute to risk assessments of chemical carcinogens across all sectors (drugs, industrial chemicals, pesticides, food additives, etc.). In the resulting risk assessment documentation, the framework analysis would be appropriately positioned within the hazard characterization section. In the absence of adequate epidemiological data, it may be regarded as an essential component in any discussion of human relevance, dose–response relationships, and risk characterization. It is also envisaged that the framework will be useful to both regulators and researchers in identifying research needs based on clear delineation of data gaps and inconsistencies.

MOA analysis can be used to establish either that a compound has an MOA that has been described previously or that it has a novel MOA. Thus, the output of an MOA analysis may serve to support the evaluation of a specific compound or contribute to the generation of a novel MOA. In the former, chemical-specific data play a vital role in the concordance analysis for human relevance. In the latter, it will be important to identify which events are key to the biological processes that represent the MOA.

Thus, an MOA comprising the same set of key events may apply to many different compounds. The evidence necessary to establish that a specific MOA is responsible for a given carcinogenic response will be substantial the first time such an MOA is proposed. As subsequent compounds are found to share this MOA, the "barrier" to acceptance will be lower, although it will always be necessary to establish rigorously that the key events comprising the MOA occur and that they fulfil the criteria described below. It will also be important to exclude other possible MOAs.

Scientific peer participation is a prerequisite for the development and acceptance of a novel postulated MOA. Peer participation includes both peer involvement in the development of an MOA and peer review by scientists who are independent of the process of development of the MOA. Publication in the scientific literature and presentation and discussion at scientific meetings and workshops constitute peer involvement that contributes to acceptance of an MOA by the scientific community.

While acceptance does not necessarily mean unanimity, most of the scientists reviewing an MOA analysis should agree that the relevant scientific information has been identified and appropriately analysed, that "key events" have been identified and are supported by the information presented, that their relationship to carcinogenesis has been clearly established in the hypothesized MOA, and that alternative MOAs have been considered and rejected.

As knowledge advances, the characterization of an MOA will change. Additional key events may be identified, and others may be refined or even dropped. Nevertheless, significant changes to the key events also need some general acceptance, through peer review, such as described above.

Update of framework guidelines

In development of the IPCS HRF, the 2001 animal MOA Framework text has been updated, and this revised version is presented here.

Introduction to framework analysis

This section describes the cancer end-point or end-points that have been observed and identifies which of these are addressed in the analysis. Prior to embarking on a framework analysis, there needs to be careful evaluation of the weight of evidence for a carcinogenic response in experimental animals. The nature of the framework is such that only one MOA is analysed at a time; hence, for example, different tumour types associated with chemical treatment, even if recorded in the same animals, will require separate framework analyses to discern each tumour's MOA. However, in considering the pathogenesis of a single type of tumour, it should be recognized that it is possible that a chemical could induce that tumour type by more than one MOA. Hence, it might be necessary to undertake an analysis of more than one MOA for the same tumour type for a single chemical. Consistent with species- and tissue-specific variation in metabolic activation and detoxication, there is often only poor site concordance for genotoxic carcinogens. This will need to be kept in mind when comparing animal and human data. In contrast, consistent with the observation that most carcinogens acting by a non-genotoxic MOA perturb physiological processes that tend to be site specific, site concordance is reasonably assumed, at least as an initial premise in the HRF.

1. Postulated mode of action (theory of the case)

This section comprises a brief description of the sequence of events on the path to cancer for the postulated MOA of the test substance. This explanation of the sequence of events leads into the next section, which identifies the events considered "key" (i.e. necessary and measurable), given the database available for the analysis.

2. Key events

This section briefly identifies and describes the "key events"—measurable events that are critical to the induction of tumours as hypothesized in the postulated MOA. To support an association, a body of experiments needs to define and measure an event consistently. Pertinent observations include, for example, tumour response and key events in the same cell type, sites of action logically related to event(s), increased cell growth, specific biochemical events, changes in organ weight and/or histology, proliferation, perturbations in hormones or other signalling systems, receptor–ligand interactions, effects on DNA or chromosomes, and impact on cell cycle. For example, key events for tumours hypothesized to be associated with prolonged regenerative proliferation might be cytotoxicity as measured histopathologically and an increase in labelling index. As another example, key events for induction of urinary bladder tumours hypothesized to be due to formation of urinary solids composed primarily of calcium phosphate might include elevated urinary free calcium, phosphate, and pH and formation of urinary solids, followed by irritation and regenerative hyperplasia of the urothelium.

3. Concordance of dose–response relationships

This section should characterize the dose–effect/response relationships for each of the key events and for the tumour response and discuss their interrelationships, in the context of the Bradford Hill criteria. Ideally, one should be able to correlate the dose dependency of the increases in incidence of a key event with increases in incidence or severity (e.g. lesion progression) of other key events occurring later in the process, and with the ultimate tumour incidence. Comparative tabular presentation of incidence of key events and tumours is often helpful in examining dose–response. In the case of complex data sets, this is almost essential.

It is important to consider whether there are fundamental differences in the biological response (i.e. dose transitions) at different parts of the dose–response curve for tumour formation (Slikker et al., 2004). If so, key events relevant to the different parts of the dose–response curve will need to be defined and used in the framework analysis.

4. Temporal association

This section should characterize the temporal relationships for each of the key events and for the tumour response. The temporal sequence of key events leading to the tumour response should be determined. Key events should be apparent before tumour appearance and should be consistent temporally with each other; this is essential in deciding whether the data support the postulated MOA. Observations of key events at the same time as the tumours (e.g. at the end of a bioassay) do not contribute to considerations of temporal association, but can contribute to analysis in the next section. Most often, complete data sets to address the criterion of temporality are not available.

5. Strength, consistency, and specificity of association of tumour response with key events

This section should discuss the weight of evidence linking the key events, precursor lesions, and the tumour response. Stop/recovery studies showing absence or reduction of subsequent events or tumour when a key event is blocked or diminished are particularly important tests of the association. Consistent observations in a number of such studies with differing experimental designs increase that support, since different designs may reduce unknown biases or confounding. Consistency, which addresses repeatability of key events in the postulated MOA for cancer in different studies, is distinguished from coherence, however, which addresses the relationship of the postulated MOA with observations in the broader database (see point 6). Pertinent observations include tumour response and key events in the same cell type, sites of action logically related to event(s), and results from multistage studies and from stop/recovery studies.

6. Biological plausibility and coherence

One should consider whether the MOA is consistent with what is known about carcinogenesis in general (biological plausibility) and also in relation to what is known for the substance specifically (coherence). For the postulated MOA and the events that are part of it to be biologically plausible, they need to be consistent with current understanding of the biology of cancer. However, the extent to which biological plausibility can be used as a criterion against which weight of evidence is assessed may be limited due to gaps in our knowledge. Coherence, which addresses the relationship of the postulated MOA with observations in the broader database—for example, association of MOA for tumours with that for other end-points—needs to be distinguished from consistency (addressed in point 5), which addresses repeatability of key events in the postulated MOA for cancer in different studies. For coherence, likeness of the case to that for structural analogues may be informative (i.e. structure–activity analysis). Information from other compounds that share the postulated MOA may be of value, such as sex, species, and strain differences in sensitivity and their relationship to key events. Additionally, this section should consider whether the database on the agent is internally consistent in supporting the purported MOA, including that for relevant non-cancer toxicities. Some MOAs can be anticipated to evoke effects other than cancer, such as reproductive effects of certain hormonal disturbances that are carcinogenic.

7. Other modes of action

This section discusses alternative MOAs that logically present themselves in the case. If alternative MOAs are supported, they need their own framework analysis. These should be distinguished from additional components of a single MOA that likely contribute to the observed effect, since these would be addressed in the analysis of the principal MOA.

8. Uncertainties, inconsistencies, and data gaps

Uncertainties should include those related to both the biology of tumour development and those for the database on the compound of interest. Inconsistencies should be flagged and data gaps identified. For the identified data gaps, there should be some indication of whether they are critical as support for the postulated MOA.

9. Assessment of postulated mode of action

This section should include a clear statement of the outcome with an indication of the level of confidence in the postulated MOA—for example, high, moderate, or low. If a novel MOA is being proposed, this should be clearly indicated. However, if the MOA is the same as that proposed for other compounds, the extent to which the key events fit this MOA needs to be stated explicitly. Any major differences should be noted, and their implications for the MOA should be discussed.

ADDRESSING THE ISSUE OF HUMAN RELEVANCE

In 2000, an IPCS Harmonization Project Cancer Planning Work Group convened in Carshalton, United Kingdom (IPCS, 2000). (This initial IPCS working group differed in membership from the subsequent IPCS working group convened to work on the human relevance project.) Among the recommendations of that meeting was the suggestion that IPCS and the International Life Sciences Institute (ILSI) move forward together and in parallel on the development of the extension of the IPCS MOA Framework towards addressing human relevance. It was recognized that ILSI could provide much help in technical workshops. In June 2001, the ILSI Risk Science Institute (RSI) with support from the USEPA and Health Canada formed a working group to examine key issues in the use of MOA information to determine the relevance of animal tumours. These efforts have resulted in several published reports that are described below. An IPCS Cancer Working Group, convened on 3–5 March 2004 in Arlington, Virginia, USA, agreed that these reports should form the starting point for further exploration of the issue of human relevance of animal tumours by IPCS with the goal of developing a unified IPCS HRF for use of MOA information in risk assessment for regulatory and other purposes (IPCS, 2004).

To address the issue of the human relevance of the MOAs determined in animals, ILSI/RSI charged its working group with expanding the IPCS MOA Framework to include evaluation of the human relevance of a cancer MOA determined in animals. The details of the process, the case-studies, and the framework were published as a series of papers in the November 2003 issue of *Critical Reviews in Toxicology* (Cohen et al., 2003; Meek et al., 2003). These articles describe the ILSI/RSI HRF and provide guidance for its application. In addition, references to specific examples on which the framework is based are included. Several iterations of case-studies of chemicals with generally well known MOAs were used to develop the integrated framework. The intent was to provide guidance for a disciplined, transparent process evaluating the MOA in animals and each key event with respect to human relevance.

The ILSI/RSI HRF is based on three fundamental questions:

1. Is the weight of evidence sufficient to establish the mode of action (MOA) in animals?
2. Are key events in the animal MOA plausible in humans?
3. Taking into account kinetic and dynamic factors, are key events in the animal MOA plausible in humans?

Questions 2 and 3 involve qualitative and quantitative considerations, respectively, in a concordance analysis of human information in relation to the animal MOA and its key events.

These are followed by an explicit description of confidence in the evaluation, identification of specific data gaps, and the implications for risk assessment. It was emphasized by ILSI/RSI that use of this framework would form part of the hazard characterization step of the overall risk assessment process.

DEVELOPMENT OF AN IPCS HRF GUIDANCE DOCUMENT BASED ON THE IPCS MOA FRAMEWORK AND THE ILSI/RSI HRF

The 2004 IPCS Cancer Working Group discussed the type of document that would be produced as a result of its task to extend the IPCS MOA Framework to address human relevance. It was recognized that one integrated guidance document that worked as a whole would be needed to facilitate uptake and use by regulatory and other risk assessment bodies. The guidance could be supplemented by publication of the other materials generated through the process (e.g. issue papers and case-studies).

There was general agreement among working group members that the questions identified as the critical components of the ILSI/RSI HRF were important and in general appropriate for addressing the human relevance of an MOA determined in animals. However, several issues were identified that could benefit from additional clarification, development, or expansion.

These refinements of the ILSI/RSI HRF were developed through discussions of the IPCS Cancer Working Group and at a workshop convened for this purpose in Bradford, United Kingdom, on 21–23 April 2005 (IPCS, 2005). The resulting IPCS HRF is presented as an approach to answering a series of three questions, leading to a documented, logical conclusion regarding the human relevance of the MOA underlying animal tumours. The application of the guidance results in a narrative with four sections that may be incorporated into the hazard characterization of a risk assessment. The sections are as follows (see Figure 1):

1. Is the weight of evidence sufficient to establish a mode of action (MOA) in animals?
2. Can human relevance of the MOA be reasonably excluded on the basis of fundamental, qualitative differences in key events between experimental animals and humans?

3. Can human relevance of the MOA be reasonably excluded on the basis of quantitative differences in either kinetic or dynamic factors between experimental animals and humans?
4. Conclusion: Statement of confidence, analysis, and implications.

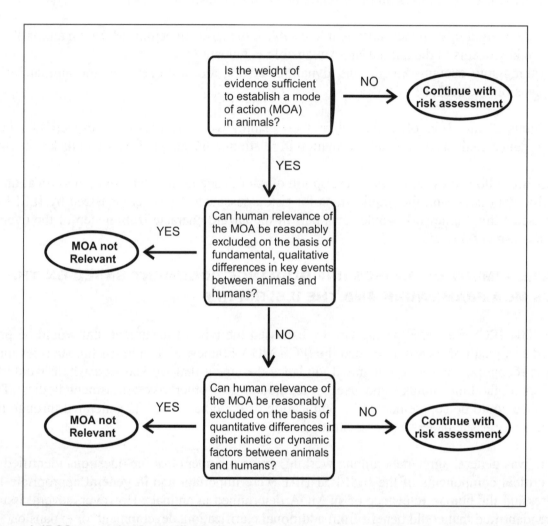

Figure 1. IPCS general scheme illustrating the main steps in evaluating the human relevance of an animal MOA for tumour formation. The questions have been designed to enable an unequivocal answer *yes* or *no*, but recognizing the need for judgement regarding sufficiency of weight of evidence. Answers leading to the left side of the diagram indicate that the weight of evidence is such that the MOA is not considered relevant to humans. Answers leading to the right side of the diagram indicate either that the weight of evidence is such that the MOA is likely to be relevant to humans or that it is not possible to reach a conclusion regarding likely relevance to humans, owing to uncertainties in the available information. In these cases, the assessment would proceed to risk characterization. It should be noted that only at this stage would human exposure be included in the evaluation.

In applying this framework for a given chemical, tumours of each animal target organ observed are evaluated independently, with the assumption that different MOAs are possible in different organs, although based on this analysis, MOAs in different tissues may be similar. Similarly, an evaluation of the likelihood of congruence between target organ(s) in different species and in humans needs to be made, based on the MOA analysis.

Is the weight of evidence sufficient to establish a mode of action (MOA) in animals?

Answering this first question in the IPCS HRF requires application of the (updated) IPCS MOA Framework described previously in this document. The steps in the MOA Framework, which are based on the Bradford Hill criteria for causality, are:

1. postulated MOA;
2. key events; associated critical parameters;
3. dose–response relationships;
4. temporal association;
5. strength, consistency, and specificity of association of key events and tumour response;
6. biological plausibility and coherence;
7. possible alternative MOAs;
8. uncertainties, inconsistencies, and data gaps;
9. conclusion about the MOA.

This process incorporates an evaluation of the weight of evidence for possible alternative MOAs at a given site and an evaluation of the overall strength of evidence supporting the MOA under consideration. Ultimately, a decision concerning the weight of evidence supporting the MOA and the level of confidence in that decision must be made. The process also identifies critically important data gaps that, when filled, would increase confidence in the proposed MOA. It is also necessary to establish whether the postulated MOA has already been described for other chemicals, in which case human relevance will already have been evaluated, or whether the proposed MOA is novel, in which case human relevance needs to be assessed de novo.

For a given chemical, the primary sources of information for evaluating an MOA are likely to be data generated for that specific chemical in the animal model in which tumours were produced. Obviously, data from other sources can and should also be used, as appropriate, along with data on chemicals with similar chemical structures, the same or similar MOAs, or both. If the MOA for a chemical is novel, considerably more data will be required to support the conclusion that it is related to the carcinogenic process of the tumours induced by that chemical than for subsequent examples of chemicals acting by the same MOA. The ILSI/RSI working group and the IPCS Bradford workshop did not address the issue of how many data are sufficient to support a specific MOA for a given chemical per se, except by way of example within the case-studies and recognition that acceptance of a novel MOA requires scientific consensus (described above). Consideration at this stage of the MOA analysis of potential variations between animals and humans also facilitates addressing subsequent steps in the framework.

Can human relevance of the MOA be reasonably excluded on the basis of fundamental, qualitative differences in key events between experimental animals and humans?

The wording of this question was changed from that in the ILSI/RSI HRF, following discussion at the IPCS workshop on the implications of a *yes* or a *no* answer to the original question. In answering the original question, only an unequivocal *no* would be sufficient to permit the conclusion that the animal MOA was not relevant to humans. Also, it was recognized that translation of the word "plausible" into other languages could be problematic. The question was therefore reworded to enable a *yes/no* answer, but qualified by the descriptor "reasonably", based on recognition that decisions about the adequacy of weight of evidence are not absolute but involve scientific judgement based on transparent analysis of the available data.

This step represents a qualitative assessment of the relevance of the MOA to human cancer potential. Listing the critical specific key events that occur in the animal MOA and directly evaluating whether each of the key events might or might not occur in humans facilitate consideration and transparent presentation of the relevant information. Presentation in tabular form, referred to as a concordance table, can be helpful in delineating the relevant information (for an example, see Meek et al., 2003, case-study 6: kidney and liver tumours associated with chloroform exposure, Table 7; McGregor et al., current document, case-study on formaldehyde, Table 3). The key events (and possibly some of the critical associated processes) are listed with the information regarding these events for the animals in which the tumour was observed. It is intended that the information in these tables be brief, since a narrative explanation is expected to accompany the table. In the right-hand column, the effect on humans for each of the key events is evaluated. An additional column for the results in a different strain, species, sex, or route of administration that does not result in tumours can be useful if information is available for comparison with the model that leads to tumours. In addition, factors may be identified that, while not key themselves, can modulate key events and so contribute to differences between species or individuals. Such factors include genetic differences in pathways of metabolism, competing pathways of metabolism, and cell proliferation induced by concurrent pathology. Any such factors identified should be noted in a footnote to the concordance table.

The evaluation of the concordance of the key events for the MOA for a given chemical in humans is an evaluation of the MOA in humans, rather than an evaluation of the specific chemical. In general, details of the initial key events are likely to be more chemical specific—for example, the enzyme induction response by phenobarbital in rodent liver, or the formation of a cytotoxic metabolite from chloroform by specific cytochrome P-450 enzymes. Later events are more generic to the MOA—for example, pleiotropic stimulation of hepatic proliferation or regenerative hyperplasia. Information that can be utilized to evaluate the key events in humans can come from in vitro and in vivo studies on the substance itself, but also can involve basic information regarding anatomy, physiology, endocrinology, genetic disorders, epidemiology, and any other information that is known regarding the key events in humans. Information concerning an evaluation of the key event in humans exposed directly to the specific chemical is frequently unavailable.

As knowledge concerning the development of cancer evolves, it may become possible to combine some MOAs on the basis of the basic biology of the processes involved, thus relying less on chemical-specific information to reach a conclusion on the human relevance of a given MOA.

In evaluating the concordance of the information in humans to that in animals, a narrative describing the weight of evidence and an evaluation of the level of confidence for the human information need to be provided. Some specific types of information that are useful include the following:

1. cancer incidences at the anatomical site and cell type of interest, including age, sex, ethnic differences, and risk factors, including chemicals and other environmental agents;
2. knowledge of the nature and function of the target site, including development, structure (gross and microscopic), and control mechanisms at the physiological, cellular, and biochemical levels;
3. human and animal disease states that provide insight concerning target organ regulation and responsiveness;
4. human and animal responses to the chemical under review or analogues following short-, intermediate-, or long-term exposure, including target organs and effects.

Obviously, a substantial amount of information is required to conclude that the given MOA is not relevant to humans. If such a conclusion is strongly supported by the data, then chemicals producing animal tumours only by that MOA would not pose a cancer hazard to humans, and no additional risk characterization for this end-point is required. Since there is no cancer hazard, there is no cancer risk for the tumour under consideration.

The question of relevance considers all groups and life stages. It is possible that the conditions under which an MOA operates occur primarily in a susceptible subpopulation or life stage—for example, in those with a pre-existing viral infection, hormonal imbalance, or disease state. Special attention is paid to whether tumours could arise from early-life exposure, considering various kinetic and dynamic aspects of development during these life stages. Any information suggesting quantitative differences in susceptibility is identified for use in risk characterization.

Can human relevance of the MOA be reasonably excluded on the basis of quantitative differences in either kinetic or dynamic factors between experimental animals and humans?

The wording of this question was changed from that in the ILSI/RSI HRF, following discussion at the IPCS workshop on the implications of a *yes* or a *no* answer to the original question. In answering the original question, only an unequivocal *no* would be sufficient to permit the conclusion that the animal MOA was not relevant to humans. The question was therefore reworded to enable a *yes/no* answer, but qualified by the descriptor "reasonably", based on recognition that decisions about the adequacy of weight of evidence are not absolute but involve judgement based on transparent analysis of the available data.

For purposes of human relevance analysis, if the experimental animal MOA is judged to be qualitatively relevant to humans, a more quantitative assessment is required that takes into account any kinetic and dynamic information that is available from both the experimental animals and humans. Such data will of necessity be both chemical and MOA specific and will include the biologically effective doses required to produce the relevant dynamic responses from which neoplasia can arise. Kinetic considerations include the nature and time course of chemical uptake, distribution, metabolism, and excretion, while dynamic considerations include the consequences of the interaction of the chemical with cells, tissues, and organs. On occasion, the biologically effective dose that would be required to create these conditions would not be possible in humans. It may also be that quantitative differences in a biological process involved in a key event—for example, the clearance of a hormone—are so great that the animal MOA is not relevant to humans. However, the IPCS workshop recognized that only infrequently is it likely that it will be possible to dismiss human relevance on the basis of quantitative differences. As with the qualitative assessment, a tabular comparison of quantitative data from the experimental animals and humans can facilitate the evaluation (for example, see Meek et al., 2003, case-study 5, thyroid tumours associated with exposure to phenobarbital, Table 6; Dellarco et al., current document, case-study on thiazopyr, Table 4). Useful comparisons can also be made with key events identified from studies of other compounds believed to induce effects by a similar MOA. For example, in the case of thiazopyr, information on the effects of phenobarbital in humans was particularly informative in evaluating the relevance of the MOA. As molecular and kinetic approaches continue to evolve, understanding of the similarities and differences of responses in animals and humans will be improved. It may become apparent that qualitative differences in a key event between an animal model and humans will be identified as being due to a specific quantitative difference, thus changing the answer to the second question (described above) to *no*.

As with question 2, if the conclusion to this question is *yes*, then chemicals producing animal tumours only by that MOA would not pose a cancer hazard to humans, and no additional risk characterization for this end-point is required.

Statement of confidence, analysis, and implications

Following the overall assessment of each of the three questions, a statement of confidence is necessary that addresses the quality and quantity of data underlying the analysis, consistency of the analysis within the framework, consistency of the database, and the nature and extent of the concordance analysis. An evaluation of alternative MOAs, using comparable analyses and rigour, is also essential. A critically important outcome of adequate consideration of the weight of the evidence for an overall MOA and the qualitative and quantitative concordance is the identification of specific data gaps that can be addressed experimentally in future investigations to increase confidence.

Infrequently, there may be conclusive epidemiological data on the cancer risk from a chemical that shares the MOA of the compound under consideration—that is, the compound does or does not cause cancer in humans. Obviously, such data would lend considerable weight to the conclusion of the human relevance evaluation. However, there may be occasions when, despite it being possible to establish an MOA in animals, there is insufficient information on the key events in humans to reach a clear conclusion on human relevance. In such circumstances, it might be possible to bridge this data gap by using epidemiological data. For example, the database on key events in humans for compounds that act like phenobarbital via activation of the constitutively active receptor (CAR) to induce hepatic tumours is incomplete. However, there are robust epidemiological data showing that exposure to phenobarbital for prolonged periods at relatively high doses does not cause cancer in humans. One possibility, therefore, is to "read across" from these findings with phenobarbital to any other compound that shares its MOA in animals in inducing rodent liver tumours and to conclude that the tumours caused by such a compound are not relevant to the risk assessment of the compound in humans (Holsapple et al., 2006). Such a conclusion would be critically dependent on the reliability of the epidemiological data and the similarity between the MOA for the chemical under test to that of the compound for which there are epidemiological data available.

In applying the framework to case-studies, it is apparent that much current research does not address key questions that would facilitate an analysis of an animal MOA or its relevance to humans. Often this has been because of lack of transparent delineation of key data gaps based on consideration of the data in analytical frameworks such as that presented here. Thus, use of the HRF can be very informative to researchers from the outset in the design of their studies.

The output of formal human relevance analysis provides information that is useful for more than just determining whether or not an end-point in animals is relevant to humans. Rather, consideration of the relevant information in a transparent, analytical framework provides much additional information that is critically important in subsequent steps in the risk characterization for relevant effects. Based on a human relevance analysis for a proposed MOA for relevant effects, it may be possible to predict, for example, site concordance or not of observed tumours in animals to humans. Application of the HRF also often provides information on relevant modulating factors that are likely to affect risk, such as hepatitis B and aflatoxin B_1 (see Cohen et al., current document, case-study on 4-aminobiphenyl). Analysis often also provides an indication of those components of a proposed MOA that may operate only over a certain dose range. If a high experimental dose of a given compound is needed to result in an obligatory step in an MOA, then the relevance to human risk becomes a matter of exposure. Thus, the exposure assessment step of the subsequent risk characterization is critical to the proper evaluation of human cancer potential. In addition, information identified during the framework analysis can prove invaluable in hazard quantification based on the key events for the MOA.

Importantly, the human relevance analysis also contributes to identification of any special subpopulations (e.g. those with genetic predisposition) who are at increased risk and often provides information relevant to consideration of relative risk at various life stages. In some cases, this may be based not on chemical-specific information but rather on inference, based on knowledge of the MOA, as to whether or not specific age groups may be at increased or decreased risk.

The data and their analysis using the framework should be reported in a transparent manner, enabling others to determine the basis of the conclusions reached with respect to the key events, the exclusion of other MOAs, and the analysis of human relevance. As the specific form of presentation will vary with the type of data available, it is not helpful to be prescriptive on how the information should be reported. However, presentation should include sufficient details on the context and thought processes to ensure transparency of the conclusions reached. The use of appropriate tables can be helpful in presenting certain data, such as comparative analysis of key events in experimental animals and humans.

Dissemination of the framework

To assist in the dissemination and application of the IPCS HRF, a database of generally accepted MOAs and informative cases should be constructed and maintained. This would comprise a series of MOAs and their associated key events, for reference by those developing framework analyses for compounds that may act by similar MOAs. The case-studies would comprise worked examples that have been analysed using the framework, to provide an indication of the relevant level of detail of the analyses and nature of the weight of evidence required to support acceptance of a proposed MOA in causing the carcinogenic response. Such cases would be particularly valuable early in the development of a new MOA.

Application of the IPCS HRF to DNA-reactive carcinogens

Because of similarities in the carcinogenic process between rodents and humans and the comparable initial interactions with DNA by DNA-reactive carcinogens, it would be expected that, in general, DNA-reactive carcinogens would be assessed as progressing to the step of "*yes*, the key events in the animal MOA could occur in humans" in the ILSI/RSI HRF, as was the case for ethylene oxide (Meek et al., 2003), and "*no*" to the equivalent step in the IPCS HRF that asks the question, "Can human relevance of the MOA be reasonably excluded on the basis of fundamental, qualitative differences in key events between experimental animals and humans?", as was the case for 4-aminobiphenyl (Cohen et al., current document). In a recent paper, Preston & Williams (2005) presented a set of key events for tumour development that provided a guide for the use of the ILSI/RSI HRF with DNA-reactive carcinogens. This guide supported the view that for most DNA-reactive chemicals, the animal MOA would be predicted to be relevant to humans. However, it was also argued that there could be exceptions and that the ILSI/RSI HRF would be a valuable tool for identifying these. Use of the ILSI/RSI HRF and the IPCS HRF can also assist in quantifying differences in key events between rodents and humans that may be of value in extrapolating risk to humans. Not all rodent DNA-reactive carcinogens have been established to be human carcinogens, as judged by the International Agency for Research on Cancer (IARC) review process. For some of these exceptions, this human–rodent difference in tumour response is attributable to lower exposure of humans to the agent or to the relative insensitivity of epidemiological studies to detect tumour responses at low exposure levels. However, there are other reasons for such differences that are based on biological considerations. For example, if a DNA-reactive carcinogen induces tumours *only* in a species-specific organ, it is possible that the animal MOA based on key events might not be relevant to humans, although available data on MOA would need to be considered to permit such a conclusion. Similarly, the generally more proficient DNA repair processes that occur in humans compared with rodents (Cortopassi & Wang, 1996; Hanawalt, 2001) or a unique pathway of bioactivation in rodents could result in there being *yes* answers to the steps in the IPCS HRF that address the queries "Can human relevance of the MOA be reasonably excluded on the basis of fundamental, qualitative differences in key events between experimental animals and humans?" and/or "Can human relevance of the MOA be reasonably excluded on the basis of quantitative differences in either kinetic or dynamic factors between experimental animals and humans?" Alternatively, the IPCS HRF could provide quantitative information on these processes for use later in the risk characterization step.

The need in applying the IPCS HRF for DNA-reactive carcinogens is to develop a set of key events that would clearly describe the cancer process and use these as the guide for establishing the human relevance of a rodent tumour MOA for any particular DNA-reactive carcinogen under consideration.

The IPCS HRF and risk assessment

Among the strengths of the framework are its flexibility, general applicability to carcinogens acting by any MOA, and the ability to explore the impact of each key event on the carcinogenic response. This includes determination of the nature of the dose–response curve, the identification and location of thresholds for individual key events, and their consequences for the overall tumour response curve. In addition, by considering the kinetic and dynamic factors involved in each key event, it may be possible to reach conclusions regarding the relevance or not of the carcinogenic response to specific subpopulations—for example, in early life, in those with particular diseases, or in those with specific polymorphisms. Alternatively, application of the framework can provide quantitative information on the differences between such groups. Application of the framework can also more generally inform the risk characterization of the chemical, even when it is concluded that the carcinogenic response per se is not relevant to humans.

As stated at the outset, MOA analysis and its human relevance counterpart are aspects of the hazard identification and characterization phases of risk assessment (National Research Council, 1983; Meek et al., 2003). Consistent with this paradigm, the human relevance case-studies referred to in the present report contribute to, but do not complete, a risk assessment for the chemicals under study. This is because a complete risk characterization requires not only evaluation of doses in the range of observations from experimental or occupational hygiene studies but also extrapolation to human exposure levels of interest in daily and lifetime activities.

Hazard characterization—and related MOA analysis—deals with the potential for harm in general terms, while the complete risk assessment puts this potential hazard into context with respect to exposure for decision-makers. Risk characterization seeks to describe the relationship between these effects and the doses to which humans are exposed in order to understand and estimate the nature and likelihood of effects in humans who are generally exposed at lower dose levels.

Understanding dose–response can have a profound effect on hazard characterization and therefore is an important component of the MOA analysis, particularly when non-linear processes or dose transitions are inherent in the relevant biology. Similarly, quantifying hazard in the context of dose informs the process of risk assessment by suggesting extrapolation models that are consistent with our understanding of the biology.

Estimating these generally lower human exposure levels is the task of the exposure analysis component of the risk assessment process. This usually involves extensive analysis of data collected from environmental media and plant and animal tissues, as well as those derived from pharmacokinetic models. This process also depends on analyses of human activity patterns and life stage and lifestyle factors that may bring about exposure. Ideally, based on this information, a range of exposure scenarios is developed for different groups (men, women, children, infants, special groups, based, for example, on ethnicity or occupation) for use in identifying populations of concern. While hazard characterization, which is largely included in the framework analysis, involves quantification (dose–response analysis), estimating external exposures and contextualizing the hazard with respect to these estimates comprise subsequent steps in the risk assessment process. For example, in the case of melamine (Meek et al., 2003, case-study 7), it was concluded that the animal MOA was potentially relevant to humans. However, recognition that bladder carcinoma formation occurred only at very high doses carried forward to the subsequent stages of the risk assessment, exposure assessment, and risk characterization. The full risk assessment established that human exposures would not achieve levels necessary to produce bladder carcinomas, by a substantial margin.

CONCLUSIONS

This IPCS HRF has been developed based on experience gained from the original 2001 IPCS MOA Framework and consideration of the 2003 ILSI/RSI human cancer relevance framework. Many aspects of these frameworks have been adopted, but a number of changes have been made to improve clarity and to introduce some elements not previously considered (e.g. sensitive subpopulations). The utility and role of the framework as an analytical tool within hazard characterization and within the overall risk assessment/characterization paradigm—that is, informing human relevance and dose–response extrapolation—have been emphasized. A number of general points and conclusions follow from the development of this framework:

1. Prior to embarking on a framework analysis, there needs to be careful evaluation of the weight of evidence for a carcinogenic response in experimental animals.
2. Peer involvement and independent review are essential prerequisites for the general acceptance and scientific defensibility of a new MOA.
3. The framework is applicable to all MOAs for carcinogens, including DNA reactivity.
4. Although human relevance is likely to be assumed for most DNA-reactive carcinogens, the human relevance analysis is a valuable approach to enhance understanding, improve characterization of the hazard and risk, and identify exceptions.
5. When dealing with a chemical that may operate through a novel MOA, the analysis is focused on the chemical and entails a detailed evaluation via the HRF. However, when a specific chemical produces a tumour response consistent with an already established and peer-reviewed MOA through which other chemicals have been shown to operate, the analysis is then focused on the established MOA and a determination of whether the chemical produces its carcinogenic effect via the same key events established for the pathway.
6. When evaluating the human relevance of a tumour response found in experimental animals, the concordance analysis of key events is for the MOA and is not necessarily a chemical-specific evaluation. Chemical-specific and generic information relevant to the carcinogenic process can be valuable in the analysis. As knowledge advances, MOAs will become less chemical specific and will be based even more on the key biological

processes involved, allowing greater generalization of human relevance from one compound to another.

7. The biological understanding and significance of the key events can inform the approach to dose–response extrapolation for cancer risk, and thus understanding of the MOA can have a profound effect on the hazard and risk characterization, particularly when non-linear processes or dose transitions are inherent in the relevant biology.

8. It is recommended that a database of generally accepted MOAs and informative case-studies be established and maintained. It should provide examples that add to the existing case-studies developed by ILSI/RSI and IPCS and that are instructive in the application of the framework analysis. This database is particularly important as experience continues to evolve in the development of MOAs of carcinogens.

9. It is important to consider potentially susceptible subgroups and different life stages in the analysis.

In conclusion, the IPCS HRF provides a rigorous and transparent approach for judging whether data support a postulated mode of carcinogenic action for a chemical and for evaluating its relevance for humans. The scientific community is encouraged to use this approach as a means to increase the use of mechanistic information in cancer risk assessment and is encouraged to provide feedback, which may lead to additional refinements in the future. The framework is of value to both the risk assessment and research communities in furthering our understanding of carcinogenic processes, in identifying critical data gaps, and in informing the design of studies related to MOAs. When a carcinogenic response is considered potentially relevant to humans, information obtained on the key events during the analysis can prove invaluable in subsequent hazard quantification of the compound. It should be possible to extend the framework to non-cancer end-points, and further work on this is recommended. Thus, application of the IPCS HRF would be an invaluable tool for harmonization across end-points.

ACKNOWLEDGEMENTS

IPCS and the authors of this paper acknowledge the numerous experts involved in the scientific meetings and workshops leading to the development of this IPCS Human Relevance Framework for Analysing the Relevance of a Cancer Mode of Action for Humans. These were expert meetings and workshops convened and conducted in accordance with procedures of the IPCS/WHO. The outcomes, including this paper, contain the collective views of an international group of experts and do not necessarily represent the decisions or the stated policy of WHO. The work was funded by donations to IPCS from a number of Member States of the World Health Assembly.

REFERENCES

Cohen M, Meek ME, Klaunig JE, Patton DE, Fenner-Crisp PA (2003) The human relevance of information on carcinogenic modes of action: An overview. *Critical Reviews in Toxicology*, **33**:581–589.

Committee on Carcinogenicity (2004) *Guidance on a strategy for the risk assessment of chemical carcinogens.* London, Department of Health.

Cortopassi GA, Wang E (1996) There is substantial agreement among interspecies estimates of DNA repair activity. *Mechanisms of Ageing and Development*, **91**:211–218.

Hanawalt PC (2001) Revisiting the rodent repairadox. *Environmental and Molecular Mutagenesis*, **38**:89–96.

Holsapple MP, Pitot HC, Cohen SM, Boobis AR, Klaunig JE, Pastoor T, Dellarco VL, Dragan YP (2006) Mode of action in relevance of rodent livers to human cancer risk. *Toxicological Sciences*, **89**:51–56.

IPCS (2000) *Scoping meeting to address the human relevance of animal modes of action in assessing cancer risk, Carshalton, United Kingdom, 8–10 November 2000.* Geneva, World Health Organization, International Programme on Chemical Safety (http://www.who.int/ipcs/methods/harmonization/areas/cancer/en/index.html).

IPCS (2004) *Report of the first meeting of the Cancer Working Group, Arlington, Virginia, USA, 3–5 March 2004.* Geneva, World Health Organization, International Programme on Chemical Safety (http://www.who.int/ipcs/methods/harmonization/areas/cancer/en/index.html).

IPCS (2005) *Record of the Cancer Framework Workshop, Bradford, United Kingdom, 21–23 April 2005.* Geneva, World Health Organization, International Programme on Chemical Safety (http://www.who.int/ipcs/methods/harmonization/areas/cancer/en/index.html).

Meek ME, Bucher JR, Cohen SM, Dellarco V, Hill RN, Lehman-McKeeman LD, Longfellow DG, Pastoor T, Seed J, Patton DE (2003) A framework for human relevance analysis of information on carcinogenic modes of action. *Critical Reviews in Toxicology*, **33**:591–653.

National Research Council (1983) *Risk assessment in the federal government. Managing the process.* Washington, DC, National Academy Press.

Preston JR, Williams GM (2005) DNA-reactive carcinogens: Mode of action and human cancer hazard. *Critical Reviews in Toxicology*, **35**:673–683.

Slikker W Jr, Andersen ME, Bogdanffy MS, Bus JS, Cohen SD, Conolly RB, David RM, Doerrer NG, Dorman DC, Gaylor DW, Hattis D, Rogers JM, Setzer RW, Swenberg JA, Wallace K (2004) Dose-dependent transitions in mechanisms of toxicity: Case studies. *Toxicology and Applied Pharmacology*, **20**:226–294.

Sonich-Mullin C, Fielder R, Wiltse J, Baetcke K, Dempsey J, Fenner-Crisp P, Grant D, Hartley M, Knaap A, Kroese D, Mangelsdorf I, Meek E, Rice J, Younes M (2001) IPCS conceptual framework for evaluating a mode of action for chemical carcinogenesis. *Regulatory Toxicology and Pharmacology*, **34**:146–152.

USEPA (1999) *Guidelines for carcinogen risk assessment (review draft).* Washington, DC, United States Environmental Protection Agency, Risk Assessment Forum (NCEA-F-0644).

USEPA (2005) *Guidelines for carcinogen risk assessment.* Washington, DC, United States Environmental Protection Agency, Risk Assessment Forum (EPA/639/P-03/001F).

THIAZOPYR AND THYROID DISRUPTION: CASE-STUDY WITHIN THE CONTEXT OF THE IPCS FRAMEWORK FOR ANALYSING THE RELEVANCE OF A CANCER MODE OF ACTION FOR HUMANS[1]

Vicki L. Dellarco, Douglas McGregor, Sir Colin Berry, Samuel M. Cohen, & Alan R. Boobis

Thiazopyr increases the incidence of male rat thyroid follicular cell tumours; however, it is not carcinogenic in mice. Thiazopyr is not genotoxic. Thiazopyr exerts its carcinogenic effect on the rat thyroid gland secondary to enhanced metabolism of thyroxine leading to hormone imbalance. The relevance of these rat tumours to human health was assessed by using the 2006 International Programme on Chemical Safety Human Relevance Framework. The postulated rodent tumour mode of action (MOA) was tested against the Bradford Hill criteria and was found to satisfy the conditions of dose and temporal concordance, biological plausibility, coherence, strength, consistency, and specificity that fits with a well established MOA for thyroid follicular cell tumours. Although the postulated MOA could theoretically operate in humans, marked quantitative differences in the inherent susceptibility for neoplasia to thyroid hormone imbalance in rats allows for the conclusion that thiazopyr does not pose a carcinogenic hazard to humans.

A number of chemical substances have been shown to induce thyroid follicular cell tumours in rats through a mode of action (MOA) that involves perturbation of thyroid hormone homeostasis via reduction of circulating thyroid hormones (Hurley et al., 1998; Capen et al., 1999; IARC, 2001). Homeostatic responses to low thyroid hormone concentrations result in a compensatory increase in the release of thyroid stimulating hormone (TSH) from the pituitary gland, which in turn stimulates the thyroid gland to increase thyroid hormone synthesis and release. Persistent elevation of TSH levels leads to thyroid follicular cell hypertrophy and hyperplasia, which, if maintained (as a result of continuous exposure to the compound), can eventually lead to neoplasia. This neoplastic MOA in rats is well accepted by the scientific community, and both the International Agency for Research on Cancer (Capen et al., 1999; IARC, 2001) and the United States Environmental Protection Agency (USEPA, 1998) have established specific guidance or policies for evaluating the human relevance of rodent thyroid follicular cell tumours.

Thiazopyr, a herbicide that induces rat thyroid follicular cell tumours by its effect on thyroid homeostasis, was the case-study used to illustrate the original 2001 International Programme on Chemical Safety (IPCS) framework for mode of carcinogenic action analysis (Sonich-Mullin et al., 2001). Thiazopyr's MOA is revisited as a case-study here to illustrate the additional guidance provided in the 2006 IPCS Human Relevance Framework (HRF) for evaluation of a neoplastic MOA for humans. This updated case-study highlights how accumulating experience with a particular MOA can make subsequent analyses less difficult. Because this case-study is based on an established MOA in which the key events have been well defined, this analysis will focus on whether thiazopyr produces the biological effects

---

[1] This article, to which WHO owns copyright, was originally published in 2006 in *Critical Reviews in Toxicology*, Volume 36, pages 793–801. It has been edited for this WHO publication and includes corrigenda.

expected of this pathway. This case-study also emphasizes the importance of understanding the basic physiological processes underlying a toxicity pathway in animals and humans. For some compounds, chemical-specific data might be critical in evaluating the key events in humans. For others, the underlying biology is sufficient to allow interpretation of the human relevance of the carcinogenic MOA, both qualitatively and quantitatively. Thiazopyr is an example of the latter. Another MOA case-study of thyroid hormone disruption and the human relevance of rat thyroid follicular cell tumours is available for phenobarbital (Lehman-McKeeman & Hill, in Meek et al., 2003).

The present MOA analysis begins with a brief summary of the available information on the carcinogenicity of thiazopyr, followed by a discussion of the experimental biochemical and histopathological data considered for this thyroid disruption MOA. It is not intended to be a comprehensive assessment of the chemical per se.

CARCINOGENICITY DATA

Human epidemiological data on the carcinogenicity of thiazopyr are not available. Thiazopyr produces effects on liver and thyroid in various laboratory species, including mice, rats, and dogs. Thiazopyr was found to induce thyroid tumours in male rats only and appears to do so by increasing the hepatic metabolism and excretion of thyroid hormones.

Chronic dietary administration of thiazopyr to mice and rats resulted primarily in thyroid follicular cell tumours in male rats but not in female rats (Naylor & McDonald, 1992; Naylor & Raju, 1992). There were no significant increases in the incidences of any tumours in either sex in the chronic study of mice treated with thiazopyr at up to 800 mg/kg in the diet (128.4 mg/kg body weight [bw] per day in males and 215.9 mg/kg bw per day in females) (Naylor & Raju, 1992). In the rat carcinogenicity study, thiazopyr (technical, 94.8% pure) was administered to male and female Sprague-Dawley (SD) rats (60 per sex per group) at dietary concentrations of 0, 1, 10, 100, 1000, or 3000 mg/kg, providing dose levels of 0, 0.04, 0.4, 4.4, 44.2, or 136.4 mg/kg bw per day for males and 0, 0.06, 0.6, 5.6, 56.3, or 177.1 mg/kg bw per day for females (Naylor & McDonald, 1992). The incidences of thyroid follicular cell adenomas and carcinomas were increased in male rats of the 1000 mg/kg (44.2 mg/kg bw per day) and 3000 mg/kg (136.4 mg/kg bw per day) groups (Table 1). It should be noted that the increase in tumour incidence in male rats is primarily accounted for by benign tumours.

POSTULATED MOA FOR THE INDUCTION OF THYROID FOLLICULAR CELL TUMOURS IN RATS

The postulated MOA for thiazopyr-induced thyroid follicular cell tumours involves the perturbation of homeostasis of the pituitary–thyroid axis by an extrathyroidal mechanism. Specifically, thiazopyr induces hepatic thyroxine (T4)-uridine diphosphate (UDP) glucuronosyltransferase (UGT) activity, leading to enhanced metabolism of T4 by conjugation and increased biliary excretion of the conjugated hormone. The result of this enhanced liver metabolism is a decrease in serum T4 (and sometimes triiodothyronine, or T3) half-life. The pituitary gland responds to a decrease in circulating serum levels of T4 by enhancing the output and serum level of TSH. Prolonged elevation of circulating TSH levels stimulates the thyroid gland to deplete its stores of thyroid hormone and continues to induce hormone production. Thus, the thyroid follicular cells enlarge (hypertrophy) and are induced to proliferate at an increased rate and to increase in number (hyperplasia). With chronic exposure, thyroid hyperplasia eventually progresses to neoplasia.

Table 1. Thyroid follicular cell tumour incidence in Sprague-Dawley male rats (2-year chronic study).

	Dose (mg/kg bw per day)[a]					
	0	*0.04*	*0.4*	*4.4*	*44.2*	*136.4[b]*
Adenomas	1/50	2/47	0/49	2/47	8/49	12/48
Carcinomas	1/50	1/47	0/49	0/47	1/49	4/48
Combined	2/50	3/47	0/49	2/47	9/49	14/48
%	(2)	(6)	(0)	(4)	(18)	(29)
P	0.000[c]	0.470	0.253	0.668	0.024*	0.001**

Note: Tumour incidences were extracted from data submitted to the USEPA Office of Pesticide Programs (Naylor & McDonald, 1992). Significance: * $P < 0.05$; ** $P < 0.01$ (statistical analyses based on Fisher's exact test).
[a] Doses in mg/kg bw per day were estimated.
[b] Two animals in the 136.4 mg/kg bw per day or 3000 mg/kg diet dose group had both benign and malignant tumours.
[c] For trend with dose.

KEY EVENTS IN EXPERIMENTAL ANIMALS

The sequence of key events in thiazopyr's mode of carcinogenic action includes:

- induction of hepatic UGT activity;
- increase in hepatic metabolism and biliary excretion of T4;
- decrease in serum T4 half-life and concentration;
- increase in circulating TSH concentration;
- cellular thyroid hypertrophy and follicular cell hyperplasia.

An evaluation follows to determine whether thiazopyr works via disruption of thyroid–pituitary status by increasing hepatic clearance of circulating thyroid hormone. Thus, based on the key events listed above, biological indicators of thiazopyr's MOA should include changes in liver metabolism, alterations in hormone levels, increases in thyroid growth, and lesion progression in the thyroid. These effects have been observed and measured in male rats in short-term and subchronic studies, and at interim and terminal sacrifices in a chronic study (Hotz et al., 1997). The dose–response and temporal analyses of the key events and tumour response are presented below.

DOSE–RESPONSE RELATIONSHIP AND CONCORDANCE

A summary of the no-observed-adverse-effect levels (NOAELs) and lowest-observed-adverse-effect levels (LOAELs) for the key effects in thiazopyr's MOA are provided in Table 2. In the 56-day study by Hotz et al. (1997), male SD rats (20 per dose) were fed diets containing thiazopyr at 0, 10, 30, 100, 300, 1000, or 3000 mg/kg (doses not measured, but estimated to be 0, 0.5, 1.5, 5, 15, 50, and 150 mg/kg bw per day) for 56 days and evaluated for the effects on liver (weights, T4-hepatic UGT activity, T4 biliary elimination), thyroid (weights, hypertrophy/hyperplasia), and hormones (serum levels of T4, T3, reverse T3, or rT3, and TSH). In this study, the effects on liver, thiazopyr's primary site of action, appear to be the most sensitive indicator of pituitary–thyroid homeostasis perturbation. Statistically significant increases in hepatic T4-UGT activity in the 50 and 150 mg/kg bw per day groups (approximately 3- and 6-fold increases in activity over controls when adjusted for liver weight, respectively) were found at the end of the 56-day treatment period. Consistent with the increase in T4-UGT activity, clearance of T4 from the blood and elimination in bile (40% increase in excretion of ^{125}I-labelled T4) were increased after 150 mg/kg bw per day of thiazopyr (only dose evaluated). Statistically significant increases in liver weight were found at 15, 50, and 150 mg/kg bw per day of thiazopyr in the 56-day study in male rats by Hotz et al. (1997). In the 2-year rat study (Naylor & McDonald, 1992), absolute liver weights were increased by 122% at 44.2 mg/kg bw per day and by 178% at 136.4 mg/kg bw per day relative to controls. There were also statistically significant increases in the incidence of liver hypertrophy at 44.2 and 136.4 mg/kg bw per day (47/61 and 52/60 versus 0/60 in controls, respectively) in the 2-year rat study.

Table 2. Summary of effects on liver, hormones, and thyroid from a 56-day study (Hotz et al., 1997) and the 2-year chronic study (Naylor & McDonald, 1992) in male rats.

Effect	NOAEL/LOAEL
Liver	
Induction of UGT	15/50 mg/kg bw per day (56-day study)
Increase in T4 biliary elimination	<150/150 mg/kg bw per day (only dose tested in 56-day study)
Increase in liver weight	5/15 mg/kg bw per day (56-day study)
	44.2/136.4 mg/kg bw per day (2-year study)
Hepatocellular hypertrophy	4.4/44.2 mg/kg bw per day (2-year study)
Hormones	
Decrease in serum T4	50/150 mg/kg bw per day (56-day study)
Increase in serum TSH	50/150 mg/kg bw per day (56-day study
Thyroid	
Increase in thyroid weight	15/50 mg/kg bw per day (56-day study)
	44.2/136.4 mg/kg bw per day (2-year study)
Increase in thyroid hyperplasia	44.2/136.4 mg/kg bw per day (2-year study)
Increase in thyroid tumours	4.4/44.2 mg/kg bw per day (2-year study)

Consistent with the enhanced hepatic clearance of T4 described above, when Hotz et al. (1997) treated male SD rats with doses of thiazopyr, statistically significant ($P \leq 0.05$) decreases in serum T4 levels (by 30%) and increases in TSH (by 60%) were found after 56 days of treatment at the highest dose tested (Table 3). T3 serum levels were non-significantly lower at 1.5 mg/kg bw per day and statistically significantly higher at 150 mg/kg bw per day after 56 days of treatment. In general, hepatic microsomal enzyme inducers appear to affect T3 less than T4; thus, T4 and TSH tend to be more reliable indicators of altered pituitary–

thyroid homeostasis (Liu et al., 1995; Hurley et al., 1998; Hood et al., 1999). In the case of thiazopyr, there appears to be a poor correlation between the doses causing the T4 and TSH effects and those causing an increased incidence of thyroid follicular cell tumours. The lowest dose of thiazopyr producing a statistically significant ($P < 0.05$) increase in thyroid follicular cell tumours in male SD rats was 44.2 mg/kg bw per day in the 2-year study, whereas the NOAEL for effects on T4 and TSH was 50 mg/kg bw per day in the 56-day study (Table 2). Generally, effects on liver enzymes/weight and pituitary–thyroid hormone concentrations would be anticipated to occur at doses at least as low as those that produce thyroid weight changes and increases in thyroid tumour incidence, given that this thyroid disruption MOA is a threshold phenomenon. This apparent discrepancy is probably not real, because neither of the doses quoted is accurate. In the 2-year study, the milligrams per kilogram body weight doses were averaged estimates for the entire study, whereas the relevant doses for comparison with the 56-day mechanistic study are those for rats of 12–20 weeks of age. These doses would have been at least 2-fold higher than those that were readily available (so the real LOAEL for neoplasia would have been about 90 mg/kg bw per day). They would also have been more relevant for neoplasia, because the critical period for hormonal perturbations (e.g. prolonged elevation of TSH) to initiate pathological changes would be early, not late, in the 2-year study. The doses calculated for the 56-day study are also likely to be inaccurate, because food intake information was not available in the publication; the doses are estimates based on assumed intakes. Having acknowledged this uncertainty, it is observed that thyroid weights were increased significantly at 50 mg/kg bw per day and liver weights were increased at 15 mg/kg bw per day, which is consistent with the liver being the initial target in thiazopyr's MOA.

Table 3. Fifty-six-day study in male rats: Hormonal effects (Hotz et al., 1997).

	Dose (mg/kg bw per day) [a]						
	0	0.5	1.5	5	15	50	150
T4 (µg/dl)	4.1 ± 0.2	4.3 ± 0.3	3.9 ± 0.2	4.1 ± 0.2	4.0 ± 0.2	4.0 ± 0.2	2.9 ± 0.1 [a]
T3 (ng/dl)	84 ± 3	82 ± 4	68 ± 2	84 ± 3	82 ± 3	91 ± 4	110 ± 6 [a]
TSH (ng/ml)	2.7 ± 0.2	3.5 ± 0.4	2.7 ± 0.1	3.1 ± 0.4	2.9 ± 0.3	3.1 ± 0.2	4.3 ± 0.4 [a]

Note: The mg/kg bw per day doses were estimated. Values are mean ± standard error of the mean; 19 or 20 animals per group.
[a] Significantly different from control with Dunnett's test after analysis of variance (ANOVA) ($P \leq 0.05$).

As stated above, prolonged TSH stimulation leads to both hypertrophy and hyperplasia of the thyroid. In the 2-year rat study, there was a poor dose correlation between thyroid hyperplasia alone and tumour incidence. While tumour incidence was increased at 44.2 mg/kg bw per day, a statistically significant increase in the incidence of hyperplasia (8/58 versus 1/60 in controls) was found only at 136.4 mg/kg bw per day. Furthermore, in the 56-day rat study, where thyroid histology was reported as follicular cell hypertrophy and hyperplasia combined, there was a significant increase in the incidence of this diagnosis at 150 mg/kg bw per day but not at lower doses (Hotz et al., 1997). There was, however, a good dose correlation between increases in thyroid weights in the 56-day study and tumour incidence in the 2-year study. Statistically significant increases in thyroid weights of 46% were found at 150 mg/kg bw per day and 25% at 50 mg/kg bw per day (Hotz et al., 1997).

TEMPORAL RELATIONSHIP

If an event (or events) is an essential element of tumorigenesis, it must precede tumour appearance. Multiple exposure time data at 7, 14, 28, 56, and 90 days are available in which male SD rats were offered diets containing thiazopyr at 3000 mg/kg (150 mg/kg bw per day) (Hotz et al., 1997). Liver weights and hepatic T4-UGT activity were increased at all observation times from the earliest time of assessment on day 7. Biliary excretion of conjugated T4 was not measured in this experiment; however, serum T4 was reduced at all observation times. Increases in circulating TSH were observed at all sampling times, although the increase was not significant at 14 days after treatment began. Increases in thyroid weight were also observed at all sampling times. Histologically, there was a time-related increase in hypertrophy/hyperplasia beginning at 14 days. In the 2-year rat study, the first thyroid adenoma was observed at week 69 at a dose of 136.4 mg/kg bw per day. Thus, there is a logical temporal response for the key events in thiazopyr-induced thyroid follicular cell tumour formation in which all key events precede tumour formation.

STRENGTH, CONSISTENCY, AND SPECIFICITY OF ASSOCIATION OF THE TUMOUR RESPONSE WITH KEY EVENTS

Strength, consistency, and specificity of the association can be established from the studies described above. The quantifiable precursor events, fundamental to the proposed MOA, are relatively consistent with the emergence of thyroid follicular cell tumours. Observation of liver weight increase and induction of hepatic T4-UGT in rats receiving the thiazopyr in the diet would be consistent with perturbation of homeostasis of the pituitary–thyroid axis by an extrathyroidal mechanism. An increase in hepatic T4-UGT activity is a step occurring before the other key biochemical changes and before thyroid follicular cell hypertrophy and hyperplasia. Thiazopyr treatment clearly results in a decrease in circulating T4 and an increase in TSH following enhanced liver metabolism of T4. Furthermore, in subchronic studies, the increases in thyroid weight and the development of hypertrophy/hyperplasia were shown to appear to a statistically significant degree under the same conditions of dose and time as the appearance and reversal of changes in thyroid hormone levels and thyroid hormone metabolism. Stop/recovery studies (Hotz et al., 1997) showed that cessation of thiazopyr dosing was followed by a return of hormone levels to control values, as well as a reduction in liver and thyroid weights and reversal of hyperplasia of thyroid follicular cells. Early dosing withdrawal would be expected to result in a reversal of hypothyroidism and of lesion progression for this non-genotoxic MOA. The only sign that was slow to reverse was the increase in thyroid weight after the longest dosing period.

BIOLOGICAL PLAUSIBILITY AND COHERENCE

There are considerable data from studies in laboratory rodents demonstrating the relationship between sustained perturbation of the hypothalamic–pituitary–thyroid axis, prolonged stimulation of the thyroid gland by TSH, and the progression of thyroid follicular cells to hypertrophy, hyperplasia, and eventually neoplasia (McClain, 1995; Hard, 1998; Hurley et al., 1998; Capen et al., 1999; IARC, 2001). Increased secretion of TSH may result via several mechanisms, including increased hepatic clearance of T4, as is the case with thiazopyr.

Circulating levels of T4 are monitored by the thyrotropic cells of the pituitary gland that are responsible for the synthesis of TSH. In the pituitary gland, T4 is metabolized by 5'-deiodinase type II to T3, which then binds to specific receptors in the cell nucleus. A decrease in T3 receptor occupancy results in stimulation of TSH synthesis and secretion. Studies in vivo have shown that injection of rats with TSH leads to reductions in thyroid follicular cell nuclear statin, a non-proliferation-specific nuclear antigen, indicating that these cells were leaving the non-dividing state to resume the cell cycle (Bayer et al., 1992). This study showed that low, repeated doses of TSH (0.25 IU per rat twice daily) produced a cumulative response in nuclear statin levels over 10 days, which returned to normal resting levels within 5 days of cessation of TSH injections. Reduction in nuclear statin is also an early event that parallels the earliest known pinocytotic response to TSH. These data are consistent with increased TSH concentrations alone causing thyroid follicular cells of rats to enter a state of pre-proliferation. Therefore, the suggestion that thiazopyr causes thyroid follicular cell neoplasms in rats by initially inducing hepatic T4-UGT is coherent with the known physiology of the hypothalamus–pituitary–thyroid dynamic control system, at least to the stage of hypertrophy and hyperplasia.

Lastly, the tumour response elicited by thiazopyr is typical of a rodent thyroid carcinogen, in that thyroid follicular cell tumours are found in male rats but not in female rats or mice. Rats tend to be more sensitive to thyroid carcinogenesis than mice, and male rats are frequently found to be more sensitive than female rats with respect to the proportion of chemicals that induce thyroid tumours (Hurley et al., 1998). In keeping with this, TSH levels are typically higher in male rats than in females (Hill et al., 1989). In addition, male rats are sometimes more prone to hepatic enzyme induction than females of the same strain, but this depends on the enzyme in question, the dose of the inducing compound, and the age of the animals (Sundseth & Waxman, 1992; Agrawal & Shapiro, 1996; Oropeza-Hernandez et al., 2003).

OTHER MODES OF ACTION

Mutagenesis is always one possible MOA to consider, but no genetic toxicity has been demonstrated for thiazopyr in the following tests:

- mutation in four strains of *Salmonella typhimurium* (Bakke, 1989a);
- mutation at the *hgpt* locus of Chinese hamster ovary cells (Li & Myers, 1989);
- micronucleus induction in bone marrow cells of mice treated in vivo (Flowers, 1990);
- unscheduled DNA synthesis induction in hepatocytes of rats treated in vivo (Bakke, 1989b).

Therefore, the available evidence indicates that mutagenesis is not an alternative MOA for thiazopyr.

Additional effects on the hypothalamic–pituitary–thyroid axis and disruption of other pathways of thyroid hormone metabolism are other possibilities for altering thyroid homeostasis. These variations would not differ in any fundamental way from the one that has been proposed for thiazopyr, in that all would lead to prolonged TSH stimulation with continuous exposure.

UNCERTAINTIES, INCONSISTENCIES, AND DATA GAPS

There appears to be a lack of dose concordance for thyroid tumours and hormone changes, but this is likely to be due to inaccuracies in the milligrams per kilogram body weight doses compared—which either were estimated (versus calculated on the basis of food consumption and body weight data) and cover an early period in the life of rats or were averages for the whole duration of the experiment—as well as experimental variability.

ASSESSMENT OF POSTULATED MODE OF ACTION

The data presented are judged, with a moderately high degree of confidence, to be adequate to explain the development of thyroid follicular cell tumours in male rats following chronic dietary exposure to thiazopyr. Thiazopyr clearly increased liver weights (i.e. the initial target organ) at doses lower than those causing tumours and enhanced thyroid growth (i.e. increased thyroid weights) at the lowest tumorigenic dose.

Human applicability of the proposed MOA

The IPCS HRF, which was developed from the Risk Science Institute/International Life Sciences Institute "Human Relevance Framework" (Meek et al., 2003) and modified based on discussions by the IPCS Cancer Working Group (Boobis et al., current document), presents a four-part approach to addressing a series of three questions and leading to a documented, logical conclusion regarding the human relevance of the MOA underlying animal tumours.

1. Is the weight of evidence sufficient to establish a mode of action (MOA) in animals? As described in detail above, there is clear evidence that thiazopyr alters thyroid homeostasis by UGT induction, by reducing serum T4 levels and consequently elevating serum TSH.

2. Can human relevance of the MOA be reasonably excluded on the basis of fundamental, qualitative differences in key events between experimental animals and humans? The current understanding of the regulation of thyroid hormone homeostasis in humans and of the role of increased TSH levels (as a result of altered thyroid homeostasis) as a risk factor for thyroid cancer was considered in order to assess the human relevance of the key events in thiazopyr's animal mode of carcinogenic action. Although there are substantial quantitative dynamic differences (discussed below), the fundamental mechanisms involved in the function and regulation of the hypothalamic–pituitary–thyroid axis in rats are qualitatively similar to those in humans (Bianco et al., 2002). Therefore, an agent that decreases T4 levels in rats could likewise reduce T4 in humans; this, in turn, could potentially lead to an increase in TSH levels. There are data showing that rodents and humans respond in a similar fashion to perturbations of pituitary–thyroid function. For example, it is well known that iodine deficiency, which readily leads to decreased thyroid hormone levels, stimulates thyroid cell proliferation in humans, leading to goitre. If left untreated, iodine deficiency may lead to tumour formation, albeit rarely (Thomas & Williams, 1999). Although there is no evidence of increased susceptibility to thyroid cancer, a number of pharmaceuticals (e.g. propylthiouracil, lithium, amiodarone, iopanoic acid) that disrupt thyroid homeostasis by acting directly on the thyroid gland (e.g. by inhibiting hormone synthesis or release or by blocking the conversion of T4 to T3) are known to lead to hypothyroidism and increases in TSH in humans (Ron et al., 1987).

In contrast to rats, no increases in TSH levels have been found in humans following exposure to agents that induce hepatic microsomal enzymes and reduce circulating T4 levels (discussed in Lehman-McKeeman & Hill, in Meek et al., 2003). For example, the pharmaceutical compounds phenytoin, rifampin, and carbamazepine induce hepatic microsomal enzymes, including UGT, and reduce circulating T4 levels, but TSH levels are unchanged (Curran & DeGroot, 1991); agents that produce thyroid tumours in rats by increasing glucuronidation and biliary excretion of T4 at high experimental doses (e.g. omeprazole, lansoprazole, and pantoprazole) produce no changes in thyroid hormones at clinical doses in humans (Masubuchi et al., 1997). Thus, there appears to be a substantial difference in the dose–response relationship for altered homeostasis of the pituitary–thyroid axis in rats compared with humans. As discussed below, this observation is due to quantitative dynamic differences between rats and humans in the basic physiological processes underlying pituitary–thyroid function.

3. Can human relevance of the MOA be reasonably excluded on the basis of quantitative differences in either kinetic or dynamic factors between experimental animals and humans? Thiazopyr does not target the thyroid directly. Rather, its primary effect is on hepatic metabolizing enzymes, and the increase in metabolic activity indirectly increases the systemic clearance of T4, leading to the hypothyroid state and the compensatory increase in TSH found in rats. Although there are no chemical-specific data on the potential for thiazopyr to disrupt thyroid hormone homeostasis in humans, a number of other microsomal enzyme inducers have been extensively studied, such as phenobarbital (Lehman-McKeeman & Hill, in Meek et al., 2003). As discussed above, agents that produce hypothyroidism by altering hepatic clearance of T4 do not appear to result in elevated TSH levels in humans. Presumably, TSH is not increased because a critical reduction of T4 is not reached.

There are several important physiological and biochemical differences between rats and humans related to thyroid function. Rats have a smaller reserve capacity of thyroid hormones when compared with humans. The rat has a much shorter thyroid hormone half-life than humans. The half-life of T4 is about 12 h in rats compared with 5–9 days in humans (Dohler et al., 1979). The shorter half-life in rats is likely related to the absence of a high affinity binding globulin for T4 that is present in humans (Hill et al., 1989). In rats, the increased clearance contributes to the need for a higher rate of production of T4 (per unit of body weight) to maintain normal levels of T4. In contrast, in humans, the binding of thyroid hormone to this globulin accounts for a slower metabolic degradation and clearance, which in turn result in the thyroid gland being less active than in rats. The constitutive TSH levels are approximately 25 times higher in rats than in humans, reflecting the higher activity of the pituitary–thyroid axis in rats (Dohler et al., 1979; McClain, 1992). Therefore, humans are quantitatively less sensitive than rats to agents that reduce T4 and lead to elevated TSH. There is no increased risk of thyroid tumour development if TSH is not elevated.

Another difference of rats compared with humans is the histological appearance of the thyroid. This histological difference is related to the higher rate of production of T4 to maintain a consistent serum concentration, thus making the rat thyroid more "functionally active" than that of primates, including humans (McClain, 1995). More of the follicular epithelium in the rat is stimulated to synthesize thyroglobulin, and therefore more of the follicular cells are tall cuboidal and appear to be active in synthesis. In contrast, more of the follicular cells in humans tend to be short cuboidal or almost squamous in appearance, suggesting they are quiescent. Because rat follicular cells are already generally active, under stimulation from TSH, they will respond with hyperplasia more readily than human follicular cells. Because of the greater storage capability of the human thyroid and the greater numbers of cells in a quiescent state, human thyroid follicular cells will be roused from their quiescent state to synthesize and secrete additional thyroid hormone without the need for a hyperplastic response to re-establish homeostasis. Therefore, the primary response in the human thyroid gland would be thyroglobulin reabsorption and cellular hypertrophy rather than hyperplasia. In short, there is much greater buffering capacity in the biochemistry of the human than the rat thyroid.

Even though certain agents can cause a reduction in thyroid hormone levels in humans, there is no clear evidence that these agents increase susceptibility to thyroid cancer (Ron et al., 1987). For example, epidemiological studies with phenobarbital do not show any increased risk of thyroid cancer (Olsen et al., 1993). Studies of individuals with conditions that would lead to elevated TSH (patients with Graves disease or goitre) indicate that the occurrence of thyroid cancer is rare in these circumstances (e.g. Mazzaferri, 2000; Gabriele et al., 2003). A study of environmental and heritable causes of cancer among 9.6 million individuals, using the nationwide Swedish Family-Cancer Database, found that the environment did not appear to play a principal causative role in thyroid cancer (Lichtenstein & Hemminki, 2002). The only known human thyroid carcinogen is radiation, a mutagenic exposure.

As summarized in Table 4, there is sufficient evidence in the general literature on the biochemical and physiological differences in thyroid function to indicate differences in tumour susceptibility between rats and humans. In contrast to humans, rats are very susceptible to thyroid neoplasia secondary to hypothyroidism. In particular, modest changes in thyroid hormone homeostasis will promote tumour formation in rats. Thus, thyroid tumours induced by thiazopyr involving increased hepatic clearance of hormone and altered homeostasis of the pituitary–thyroid axis in rodents are considered not relevant to humans, based on quantitative dynamic differences.

4. Conclusion: statement of confidence, analysis, and implications. There is sufficient experimental evidence to establish a thyroid disruption MOA for thiazopyr-induced thyroid follicular cell tumours in rats. Although thiazopyr may potentially result in hypothyroidism in humans, there is sufficient quantitative evidence on the basic physiological processes in the general literature to conclude that thyroid tumours induced by a process involving increased hepatic clearance of thyroid hormone and altered homeostasis of the pituitary–thyroid axis in rodents is not likely to lead to an increase in susceptibility to tumour development in humans. Although there are no human data on thiazopyr, clinical data on other hepatic microsomal enzyme inducers were critical to this human relevance analysis. The general literature provided sufficient evidence to show that unlike in the rat, decreased T4 levels typically show no evidence of compensatory increases in TSH levels in humans. There is also cellular and biochemical evidence that the rat pituitary–thyroid axis is much more sensitive than that in humans to such perturbations. This sensitivity is likely the result of the rapid turnover of T4 in rats coupled with the higher demand for TSH to maintain thyroid activity.

Table 4. A comparison of key events in rats and humans.

Key event	Evidence in rats	Evidence in humans
Increased hepatic clearance of T4	In short-term and chronic rat studies, the liver is found to be the most sensitive target, and evidence of increased T4 hepatic clearance is provided by studies on T4-hepatic UGT activity, T4 half-life, T4 biliary elimination, liver weights, and hypertrophy.	No data available for thiazopyr, but microsomal enzyme induction is plausible.
Decreased serum T4	Direct experimental evidence.	No data available for thiazopyr, but plausible given that other microsomal enzyme inducers have been shown to reduce T4 in humans.
Increased TSH levels	Direct experimental evidence.	No data available for thiazopyr, but other microsomal enzyme inducers have not been shown to increase TSH levels even when T4 is decreased.
Increased TSH increases thyroid cell proliferation and tumour formation	Direct experimental evidence.	Induction of thyroid follicular cell tumours secondary to hypothyroidism is remote in humans, given the quantitative differences in thyroid function/homeostasis. Occurrence of thyroid cancer is rare even in severely hypothyroid individuals.

IMPLICATIONS OF THE IPCS HRF

The thiazopyr example is an illustration of an induced tumour response consistent with an MOA that has been previously defined and established. Thus, addressing the first question in the framework analysis, "Is the weight of evidence sufficient to establish a mode of action (MOA) in animals?", became a determination of whether the data set on the chemical conforms to the same key events defined for the pathway of interest. This example further demonstrates how data on the basic understanding of the biological processes involved in the MOA provide an important means to compare the rodent and human key events. Thus, this generic human information was essential to evaluating the qualitative and quantitative differences between experimental animals and humans in addressing the plausibility of the cancer MOA for humans (i.e. questions 2 and 3 in the HRF).

REFERENCES

Agrawal AK, Shapiro BH (1996) Phenobarbital induction of hepatic CYP2B1 and CYP2B2: Pretranscriptional and post-transcriptional effects of gender, adult age, and phenobarbital dose. *Molecular Pharmacology*, **49**(3):523–531.

Bakke JP (1989a) *Ames/*Salmonella *mutagenicity assay with MON 13200: Study No. ML-88-191/EHL No. 88124.* Testing facility: Monsanto's Environmental Health Laboratory, St. Louis, MO. Submitted by Monsanto, St. Louis, MO (MRID No. 42275535).

Bakke JP (1989b) *Evaluation of MON 13200 to induce unscheduled DNA synthesis in the in vitro hepatocyte DNA repair assay in the male F-344 rat: Study No. SR-88-204/SRI No. LSC 6327.* Testing facility: SRI International, Menlo Park, CA. Submitted by Monsanto, St. Louis, MO (MRID No. 42275538).

Bayer I, Mitmaker B, Gordon PH, Wang E (1992) Modulation of nuclear statin expression in rat thyroid follicle cell following administration of thyroid stimulating hormone. *Journal of Cellular Physiology*, **150**:276–282.

Bianco AC, Salvatore D, Gereben B, Berry MJ, Larsen PR (2002) Biochemistry, cellular and molecular biology, and physiological roles of the iodothyronine selenodeiodinases. *Endocrine Reviews*, **23**(1):38–89.

Capen CC, Dybing E, Rice JM, Wilbourn JD, eds (1999) *Species differences in thyroid, kidney and urinary bladder carcinogenesis.* Lyon, International Agency for Research on Cancer (IARC Scientific Publications No. 147).

Curran PG, DeGroot LJ (1991) The effect of hepatic enzyme-inducing drugs on thyroid hormones and the thyroid gland. *Endocrine Reviews*, **12**:135–150.

Dohler KD, Wong CC, Von Zur Muhlen A (1979) The rat as a model for the study of drug effects on thyroid function: Consideration of methodological problems. *Pharmacology and Therapeutics*, **5**:305–318.

Flowers LJ (1990) *Micronucleus assay with MON 13200: ML-88-390/EHL Study No. 88230.* Testing facility: Monsanto's Environmental Health Laboratory, St. Louis, MO. Submitted by Monsanto, St. Louis, MO (MRID No. 42275537).

Gabriele R, Letizia C, Borghese M, De Toma G, Celia M, Izzo L, Cavalla A (2003) Thyroid cancer in patients with hyperthyroidism. *Hormone Research*, **60**(2):79–83.

Hard GC (1998) Recent developments in the investigation of thyroid regulation and thyroid carcinogenesis. *Environmental Health Perspectives*, **106**(8):1–21.

Hill RN, Erdreich LS, Paynter OE, Roberts PA, Rosenthal SL, Wilkinson CF (1989) Thyroid follicular cell carcinogenesis. *Fundamental and Applied Toxicology*, **12**(4):629–697.

Hood A, Liu YP, Gattone VH 2nd, Klaassen CD (1999) Sensitivity of thyroid gland growth to thyroid stimulating hormone (TSH) in rats treated with antithyroid drugs. *Toxicological Sciences*, **49**:263–271.

Hotz KJ, Wilson AG, Thake DC, Roloff MV, Capen CC, Kronenberg JM, Brewster DW (1997) Mechanism of thiazopyr-induced effects on thyroid hormone homeostasis in male Sprague-Dawley rats. *Toxicology and Applied Pharmacology*, **142**:133–142.

Hurley PM, Hill RN, Whiting RJ (1998) Mode of carcinogenic action of pesticides inducing thyroid follicular-cell tumors in rodents. *Environmental Health Perspectives*, **106**(8):437–445.

IARC (2001) *Some thyrotropic agents*. Lyon, International Agency for Research on Cancer, 763 pp. (IARC Monographs on the Evaluation of Carcinogenic Risks to Humans, Vol. 79).

Li AP, Myers CA (1989) *CHO/HGPRST gene mutation assay with MON 13200: Study No. ML-88-382/EHL No. 88071*. Testing facility: Monsanto's Environmental Health Laboratory, St. Louis, MO. Submitted by Monsanto, St. Louis, MO (MRID No. 42275536).

Lichtenstein CK, Hemminki K (2002) Environmental and heritable cause of cancer among 9.6 million individuals in the Swedish Family-Cancer Database. *International Journal of Cancer*, **1099**(2):260–266.

Liu J, Liu Y, Barter RA, Klaassen CD (1995) Alteration of thyroid homeostasis by UDP-glucuronosyltransferase inducers in rats: A dose–response study. *Journal of Pharmacology and Experimental Therapeutics*, **273**:977–985.

Masubuchi N, Hakusui H, Okazaki O (1997) Effects of proton pump inhibitors on thyroid hormone metabolism in rats: A comparison of UDP-glucuronyltransferase induction. *Biochemical Pharmacology*, **54**(11):1225–1231.

Mazzaferri EL (2000) Thyroid cancer and Graves' disease: The controversy ten years later. *Endocrine Practice*, **6**:221–225.

McClain RM (1992) Thyroid gland neoplasia: Non-genotoxic mechanisms. *Toxicology Letters*, **64/65**:397–408.

McClain RM (1995) Mechanistic considerations for the relevance of animal data on thyroid neoplasia to human risk assessment. *Mutation Research*, **333**(1–2):131–142.

Meek ME, Bucher JR, Cohen SM, Dellarco V, Hill RN, Lehman-McKeeman LD, Longfellow DG, Pastoor T, Seed J, Patton DE (2003) A framework for human relevance analysis of information on carcinogenic modes of action. *Critical Reviews in Toxicology*, **33**(6):591–654.

Naylor MW, McDonald MM (1992) *Chronic study of MON 13200 administered in feed to albino rats. Project No. ML-88-247/EHL 88148.* Testing facility: Monsanto Company, The Agricultural Group, Environmental Health Laboratory, St. Louis, MO. Submitted by Monsanto Agricultural Company, St. Louis, MO (MRID No. 426197-24).

Naylor MW, Raju NR (1992) *Chronic study of MON 13200 administered in feed to albino mice. Project No. ML-88-248/EHL 88147.* Testing facility: Monsanto Company, The Agricultural Group, Environmental Health Laboratory, St. Louis, MO. Submitted by Monsanto Agricultural Company, St. Louis, MO (MRID No. 426197-23).

Olsen JH, Wallin H, Boice JD, Rask K, Schulgen G, Fraumaen FF Jr (1993) Phenobarbital, drug metabolism and human cancer. *Cancer Epidemiology, Biomarkers and Prevention,* **5**:449–452.

Oropeza-Hernandez LF, Lopez-Romero R, Albores A (2003) Hepatic CYP1A, 2B, 2C, 2E and 3A regulation by methoxychlor in male and female rats. *Toxicology Letters,* **144**(1):93–103.

Ron E, Kleinerman RA, Boice JD, LiVolsi VA, Flannery JT, Fraumeni JF Jr (1987) A population-based case–control study of thyroid cancer. *Journal of the National Cancer Institute,* **79**:1–12.

Sonich-Mullin C, Fielder R, Wiltse J, Baetcke K, Dempsey J, Fenner-Crisp P, Grant D, Hartley M, Knaap A, Kroese D, Mangelsdorf I, Meek E, Rice JM, Younes M (2001) IPCS conceptual framework for evaluating a mode of action for chemical carcinogenesis. *Regulatory Toxicology and Pharmacology,* **34**:146–152.

Sundseth SS, Waxman DJ (1992) Sex-dependent expression and clofibrate inducibility of cytochrome P450 4A fatty acid omega-hydroxylases. Male specificity of liver and kidney CYP4A2 mRNA and tissue-specific regulation by growth hormone and testosterone. *Journal of Biological Chemistry,* **267**(6):3915–3921.

Thomas GA, Williams ED (1999) Thyroid stimulating hormone (TSH)-associated follicular hypertrophy and hyperplasia as a mechanism of thyroid carcinogenesis in mice and rats. In: Capen CC, Dybing E, Rice JM, Wilbourn JD, eds. *Species differences in thyroid gland, kidney and urinary bladder carcinogenesis.* Lyon, International Agency for Research on Cancer, pp. 45–59 (IARC Scientific Publications No. 147).

USEPA (1998) *Assessment of thyroid follicular cell tumors.* Washington, DC, United States Environmental Protection Agency, Office of Research and Development, Risk Assessment Forum (EPA/630/R-97/002; http://cfpub.epa.gov/ncea/raf/recordisplay.cfm?deid=13102; accessed 22 November 2004).

4-AMINOBIPHENYL AND DNA REACTIVITY: CASE-STUDY WITHIN THE CONTEXT OF THE IPCS FRAMEWORK FOR ANALYSING THE RELEVANCE OF A CANCER MODE OF ACTION FOR HUMANS[1]

Samuel M. Cohen, Alan R. Boobis, M.E. (Bette) Meek, R. Julian Preston, &
Douglas B. McGregor

The International Programme on Chemical Safety (IPCS) Human Relevance Framework (HRF) was evaluated for a DNA-reactive (genotoxic) carcinogen, 4-aminobiphenyl, based on a wealth of data in animals and humans. The mode of action (MOA) involves metabolic activation by *N*-hydroxylation, followed by *N*-esterification leading to the formation of a reactive electrophile, which binds covalently to DNA, principally to deoxyguanosine, leading to an increased rate of DNA mutations and ultimately to the development of cancer. In humans and dogs, the urinary bladder urothelium is the target organ, whereas in mice, it is the bladder and liver; in other species, other tissues can be involved. Differences in organ specificity are thought to be due to differences in metabolic activation versus inactivation. Based on qualitative and quantitative considerations, the MOA is possible in humans. Other biological processes, such as toxicity and regenerative proliferation, can significantly influence the dose–response of 4-aminobiphenyl-induced tumours. Based on the IPCS HRF, 4-aminobiphenyl would be predicted to be a carcinogen in humans, and this is corroborated by extensive epidemiological evidence. The IPCS HRF is useful in evaluating DNA-reactive carcinogens.

4-Aminobiphenyl is carcinogenic when administered to several species by a variety of routes (IARC, 1972, 1986, 1987). It was selected as a chemical for a case-study for the International Programme on Chemical Safety (IPCS) Human Relevance Framework (HRF) as a representative DNA-reactive carcinogen because of its established mode of action (MOA) in animal models, based on substantial data available evaluating its metabolic activation, DNA reactivity, genotoxicity, and carcinogenicity. It is also similar to numerous known animal and human carcinogens belonging to the chemical class of aromatic amines (structure–activity relationships), and there are extensive epidemiological, metabolic, and biochemical data in humans. This case-study illustrates the nature of data that are helpful in delineating MOAs for DNA-reactive carcinogens. Distinction between modulating factors and key events in an MOA analysis is also presented.

Based on the strong animal evidence and extensive epidemiological data, the International Agency for Research on Cancer (IARC) has classified 4-aminobiphenyl as a known human carcinogen (IARC, 1972, 1987). Although initially identified as a human urinary bladder carcinogen in individuals exposed to high levels occupationally, it has subsequently been demonstrated as a major component of cigarette smoke, leading to an increased risk of urinary bladder cancer in cigarette smokers (Del Santo et al., 1991; Curigliano et al., 1996). Additional research has shown that it is a ubiquitous environmental chemical occurring naturally when organic material containing nitrogen undergoes combustion.

---

[1] This article, to which WHO owns copyright, was originally published in 2006 in *Critical Reviews in Toxicology*, Volume 36, pages 803–819. It has been edited for this WHO publication and includes corrigenda.

CARCINOGENICITY OF 4-AMINOBIPHENYL IN ANIMALS

Experimental studies indicate that 4-aminobiphenyl is carcinogenic in mice, rats, rabbits, and dogs, although significant target tissue differences and susceptibility have been observed (IARC, 1972). By most routes of exposure, 4-aminobiphenyl is primarily a carcinogen of the liver and, to a lesser extent, the urinary bladder in mice, whereas in dogs (and humans), the urinary bladder appears to be the target organ. Many of the studies were conducted a number of years ago, and published accounts include only limited details. In addition, potential precursor lesions at interim periods were rarely documented, and none of the studies included protocols, such as stop/recovery, which might be informative in the context of MOA. Nonetheless, results indicate clear species and individual differences in response (e.g. Block et al., 1978), characteristic of MOAs entailing competing metabolic activation and deactivation processes (Table 1).

Table 1. Carcinogenicity studies of 4-aminobiphenyl in various species.

Species	Route/dose	Incidence	Comment	Reference
Mice	Gavage; 1 mg/week for 38 weeks	Bladder carcinomas in 2/12 mice surviving to 90 weeks		Clayson et al. (1965)
Mice	Gavage; 0 or 1.5 mg/week for 52 weeks	Bladder carcinomas in 1/21 exposed males vs 0/19 in controls; increased incidence of hepatomas in males and females		Clayson et al. (1967)
Mice	Subcutaneous injection of 200 µg for up to 52 weeks	Hepatomas in 19/20 males and 6/23 females after 48–52 weeks		Gorrod et al. (1968)
Mice (BALB/cStCrlfC3Hf/Nctr)	0–220 mg/l in drinking-water (males), 0–300 mg/l (females), for up to 96 weeks	Significant increases in urinary bladder carcinomas (males only), hepatocellular carcinomas (females only), and angiosarcomas (males and females)	Hyperplasia of the bladder in most mice of both sexes receiving 75 mg/l (females) and 55 mg/l (males) or greater, but none in controls	Schieferstein et al. (1985)
Mice (newborn B6C3F1)	Different regimens; injected prior to weaning	Liver tumours		Dooley et al. (1988, 1992); Von Tungeln et al. (1996); Parsons et al. (2005)
Rats	Subcutaneous injection in arachis oil of total dose of 3.6–5.8 g/kg bw	Mammary and intestinal tumours		Walpole et al. (1952)

Table 1 (Contd)

Species	Route/dose	Incidence	Comment	Reference
Rabbits	Oral administration of unspecified dose	Bladder papillomas in 1 animal and carcinomas in 3 animals	Earliest carcinoma observed 4 years after start of treatment	Bonser (1962)
Dogs (2)	Gelatin capsules 6 times weekly for life for a total dose of 30 or 34 g	Carcinoma of the bladders appeared in 33 months		Walpole et al. (1954)
Dogs	Gelatin capsules 0.3 g 3 times weekly (total dose: 94.5–144 g per dog)	Bladder carcinomas after 21–34 months		Deichmann et al. (1958)
Dogs (6)	1.0 mg/kg bw 5 times weekly for 34 or 37 months (total dose 5.5–7.0 g per dog)	3 bladder papillomas and 3 bladder carcinomas (transitional cell type)		Deichmann et al. (1965)
Dogs	Single dose	Ineffective in inducing bladder tumours over a 5-year period		Deichmann & MacDonald (1968)
Dogs (24 beagles)	Oral administration 5 days/week for 3 years	Negative or minimal disease in 4 dogs, with no neoplasia in 2; neoplasia developed slowly in 11 dogs, while a rapidly progressive pattern was observed in the remaining 9 dogs		Block et al. (1978)

bw, body weight

Following its oral administration by gavage (1 mg per mouse per week for 38 weeks), 2/12 mice surviving to 90 weeks developed bladder carcinoma (Clayson et al., 1965). In a separate but similar experiment, dosing mice with 1.5 mg of 4-aminobiphenyl for 52 weeks resulted in bladder carcinoma in 1/21 male mice as compared with 0/19 in controls. In this experiment, the frequency of hepatomas in both male and female mice was significantly higher than that in the controls (Clayson et al., 1967). Three subcutaneous injections of mice with 200 µg of 4-aminobiphenyl produced hepatomas in 19/20 males and 6/23 females after 48–52 weeks (Gorrod et al., 1968). Oral administration of 4-aminobiphenyl in drinking-water at concentrations of up to 220 and 300 mg/l to male and female BALB/cStCrlfC3Hf/Nctr mice, respectively, for up to 96 weeks induced dose-related, significant increases in angiosarcomas (males and females), urinary bladder carcinomas (males only), and hepatocellular carcinomas (females only). Hyperplasia of the bladder was observed in most of the mice of both sexes in groups of about 118 receiving concentrations of 75 mg/l (females) and 55 mg/l (males) or greater, whereas none was reported in the control groups of similar size (Schieferstein et al., 1985). In a number of experiments, newborn B6C3F1 mice were primarily susceptible to liver carcinogenesis following 4-aminobiphenyl administration (Dooley et al., 1988, 1992; Von Tungeln et al., 1996; Parsons et al., 2005).

Daily subcutaneous injection of rats with 4-aminobiphenyl in arachis oil to a total dose of 3.6–5.8 g/kg body weight (bw) resulted in significant increases in the incidence of mammary gland and intestinal tumours (Walpole et al., 1952).

Among seven rabbits given commercial 4-aminobiphenyl orally (dose unstated), bladder papillomas were found in one and carcinomas in three animals. The earliest carcinoma was observed 4 years after the start of treatment (Bonser, 1962).

Two dogs fed 4-aminobiphenyl in gelatin capsules 6 times weekly for life (total dose per dog: 30, 34 g) developed carcinoma of the bladder in 33 months (Walpole et al., 1954). This was confirmed by similarly feeding capsules containing 4-aminobiphenyl (0.3 g per dog) 3 times weekly. Bladder carcinomas were observed after 21–34 months (total dose: 94.5–144.0 g per dog) (Deichmann et al., 1958). When the dose of 4-aminobiphenyl was reduced to 1.0 mg/kg bw and given to six dogs 5 times weekly for 34 months or 37 months (total dose: 5.5–7.0 g per dog), three bladder papillomas and three bladder carcinomas (transitional cell type) were observed (Deichmann et al., 1965). A single dose was not effective in inducing bladder tumours over a period of 5 years (Deichmann & MacDonald, 1968). Among 24 beagles that received 4-aminobiphenyl orally 5 days per week for 3 years, three basic patterns of bladder carcinogen responses were seen. Negative or minimal disease was seen in four dogs, of which two remained completely free of neoplasia. Neoplasia developed slowly in 11 dogs, while a rapidly progressive pattern was observed in the remaining 9 dogs (Block et al., 1978).

IS THE WEIGHT OF EVIDENCE SUFFICIENT TO ESTABLISH A MODE OF ACTION (MOA) IN ANIMALS?

The first question of the IPCS HRF is an evaluation of the animal MOA itself. This is based on the process delineated by the MOA Framework developed by IPCS and published in 2001 (Sonich-Mullin et al., 2001), which evolved from the Bradford Hill criteria for causality in epidemiology studies (Hill, 1965).

A. Postulated mode of action

4-Aminobiphenyl is metabolized by hepatic enzymes to *N*-hydroxy-4-aminobiphenyl, which can be *N*-esterified (*N*-acetylated, *N*-glucuronidated, or *N*-sulfated) in hepatic and other tissues (Miller et al., 1961; Kadlubar et al., 1977, 1991; Miller & Miller, 1977; Delclos et al., 1987; Chou et al., 1995) (Figure 1). *O*-Esterification and ring hydroxylation are competing enzymatic reactions leading to detoxification. Tissue and species differences in the activity of these reactions dictate, at least in part, variations in susceptibility to the carcinogenic effects of 4-aminobiphenyl and differences in organ specificity in the development of tumours. Ultimately, a reactive electrophilic nitrenium ion is formed in the target tissue following *N*-esterification, and this is capable of forming DNA adducts. The principal DNA adduct is *N*-(deoxyguanosin-8-yl)-4-aminobiphenyl (Talaska et al., 1990; Kadlubar et al., 1991; Flammang et al., 1992; Hatcher & Swaminathan, 1995, 2002). As a consequence of the

47

mutations that can result from these reactions at critical sites of critical genes, neoplastic cells eventually develop.

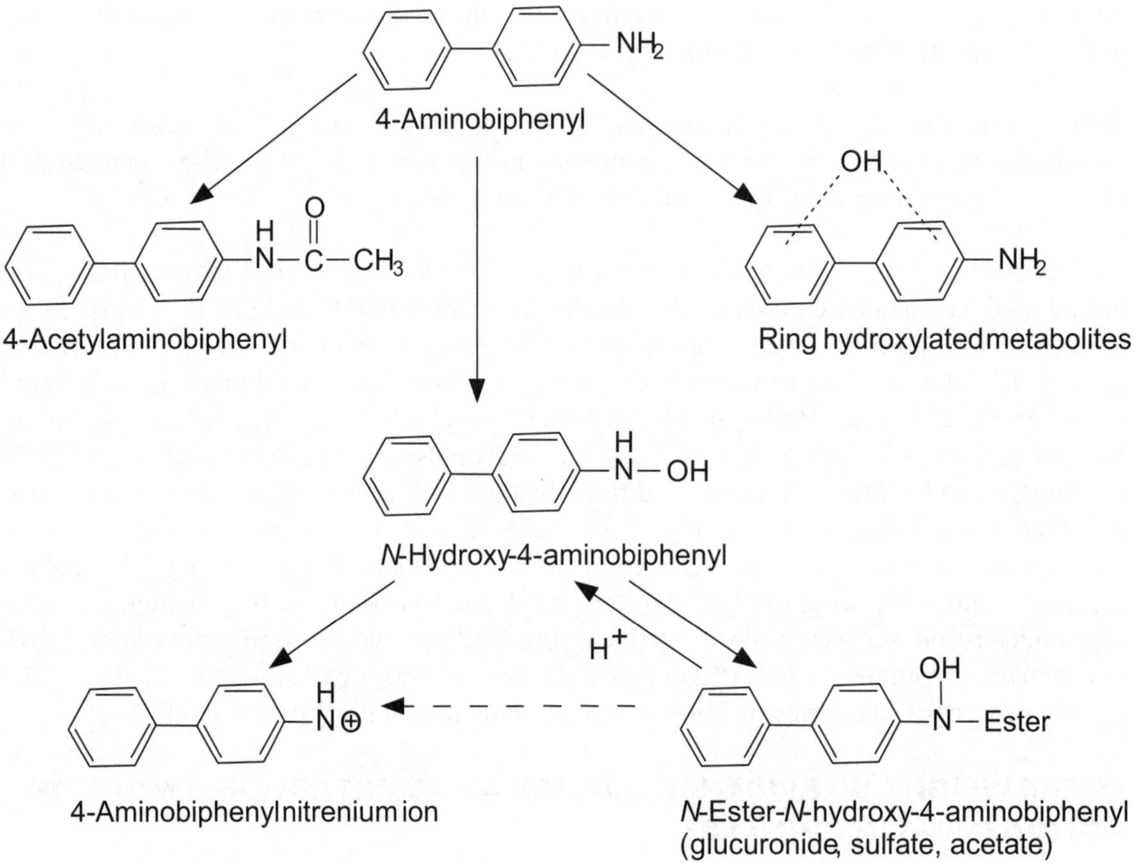

Figure 1. Metabolism of 4-aminobiphenyl

B. Key events

The major route of hepatic activation of 4-aminobiphenyl begins with its *N*-hydroxylation, catalysed, the balance of evidence indicates, by CYP1A2, at least in rats and humans (Butler et al., 1989b). In mice, there is evidence that CYP1A2 is not the only, or even the primary, form of cytochrome P-450 involved (Kimura et al., 1999). The *N*-hydroxylamine can also be produced by reaction with a variety of oxidases and peroxidases, such as by the prostaglandin synthase component of cyclo-oxygenase (Kadlubar et al., 1982). Whether any of these non-cytochrome P-450 reactions occur in vivo and are of toxicological significance remains unclear. The *N*-hydroxylamine undergoes *N*-acetylation by *N*-acetyltransferase-1 (NAT1) (Flammang & Kadlubar, 1986; Oda, 2004), resulting in an *N*-acetoxy ester that is unstable in acidic conditions, forming an arylnitrenium ion that can react directly with DNA, forming a DNA adduct at the C-8 position of guanine (Hammons et al., 1985; Flammang & Kadlubar, 1986; Hatcher & Swaminathan, 2002). Additionally, the *N*-hydroxylamine generated in liver can serve as a substrate for uridine diphosphate (UDP) glucuronosyltransferase (UGT), yielding an *N*-glucuronide conjugate that is transported to the urinary bladder (Kadlubar et al., 1977). The glucuronide can either be excreted in urine or, under acidic conditions, serve as an additional source of the *N*-hydroxylamine in the urinary bladder, following hydrolysis. There are a number of reactions that can compete with this reaction scheme, including *N*-acetylation of 4-aminobiphenyl by *N*-acetyltransferase-2 (NAT2), but the resulting arylacetamide is a poor substrate for CYP1A2, and it is considered to be primarily a detoxification reaction. As a consequence, *N*-acetylation of the parent amine is considered a deactivating process. Rates of acetylation can thus affect the balance between activation and deactivation. Humans phenotypically are either rapid or slow acetylators (Lower et al., 1979). Mouse strains exist that are analogous to human slow and rapid acetylators. Thus, C57BL/6 is a rapid acetylator strain, while A/J is a slow acetylator (Hein, 1988). Interest in these differences includes a possible explanation for interspecies, interstrain, and interindividual differences in response. As a consequence of the DNA adducts formed, mutations can be produced. The key events are summarized in Table 2.

Table 2. Key events in the carcinogenicity of 4-aminobiphenyl in animals.

1.	Metabolic activation
	a) *N*-Hydroxylation
	b) *N*-Esterification (glucuronide, acetyl, sulfate)
	c) Hydrolysis to nitrenium ion
2.	DNA adduct formation (dG-C8, dA-C8, dG-N2) in pluripotential cell of target organ
3.	DNA mutation in critical gene(s) leading to cancer
4.	Cancer

dA, deoxyadenosine; dG, deoxyguanosine

C. Dose–response relationship

In view of the fact that many of the relevant studies were conducted a number of years ago, data on concordance of dose–response for precursor lesions for tumours are restricted to hyperplasia in the mouse urinary bladder. Dogs do not develop bladder tumours after a single dose of 4-aminobiphenyl (Deichmann & MacDonald, 1968), and there do not appear to have been studies of dose–response relationships in this species following multiple exposures. In the only study in which information on the incidence of precursor lesions was reported, male BALB/c mice were treated with drinking-water containing 4-aminobiphenyl at concentrations of 0, 7, 14, 28, 55, 110, or 220 mg/l for up to 96 weeks (Schieferstein et al., 1985). These treatments were associated with bladder carcinoma incidences of 0/116, 1/117, 1/118, 0/118, 6/115, 5/118, and 23/118, respectively. The incidences in the 55 mg/l group and higher were statistically significantly higher than in controls. Female mice were exposed to drinking-water concentrations of 4-aminobiphenyl of 0, 7, 19, 38, 75, 150, and 300 mg/l. The corresponding incidences of bladder carcinomas were 0/118, 0/118, 0/119, 1/118, 0/118, 5/117, and 1/117. Incidences of hyperplasia were much higher, although severity was not indicated. In males, the incidences of hyperplasia were 0/116, 4/117, 9/118, 71/118, 108/115, 107/118, and 102/118 for doses of 0, 7, 14, 28, 55, 110, and 220 mg/l, respectively, and for females, 0/118, 0/118, 3/119, 53/119, 106/118, 97/117, and 83/117 for doses of 0, 7, 19, 38, 75, 150, and 300 mg/l, respectively. Thus, the dose–response curves for tumours and hyperplasia were sigmoidal or hockey stick-shaped. In contrast, steady-state levels of urothelial C-8 guanine DNA adducts showed a linear dose–response (Poirier et al., 1995).

In this same study (Schieferstein et al., 1985), there was no increase in the incidence of liver tumours in the males, whereas in the females, the incidences of liver tumours (adenomas and carcinomas combined) were 0/117, 0/120, 2/120, 4/119, 11/119, 17/118, and 10/117 at doses of 0, 7, 19, 38, 75, 150, and 300 mg/l, respectively. The incidence of angiosarcomas of various tissues combined was also increased at the three highest doses in males and females, although the incidences were somewhat higher in females than in males.

D. Temporal relationship

Establishing time sequences for events in a carcinogenic process is partially, but to an important extent, dependent upon the sensitivity of the available methods for their measurement. Thus, tumours must attain a size allowing their histological detection, while the measurement of mutations and DNA adducts requires not only time but sufficient tissue. Consequently, the latter are more usually studied in liver than in urinary bladder, where the paucity of tissue available in the urothelium, particularly in rodents, causes technical difficulties that have no connection with the frequency of the biochemical and biological events. The metabolism and formation of DNA adducts are early events, which can be observed within a few minutes or hours in vitro and within a day following in vivo treatment with 4-aminobiphenyl (e.g. Kadlubar et al., 1991; Swaminathan & Reznikoff, 1992; al-Atrash et al., 1995; Hatcher & Swaminathan, 1995; Doerge et al., 1999; Tsuneoka et al., 2003). Many in vivo experiments, however, continue exposure for 3–4 weeks to allow an accumulation of adducts, achieve steady-state levels, and facilitate their detection (e.g. Talaska et al., 1990; Flammang et al., 1992; Poirier & Beland, 1992; Poirier et al., 1995; Underwood et al., 1997). Mutations can also be detected within a short time in vitro, but have generally not been detected in vivo in target tissues until after several weeks or months of exposure (e.g. H-*ras* in mouse liver; Parsons et al., 2002), although this comparatively long period may not be a true reflection of when mutations first arise. In one study, mutations were detected in a Muta™Mouse urinary bladder assay 14 days after a single dose of 4-aminobiphenyl (Fletcher et al., 1998). Carcinomas and hyperplasia of the urinary bladder are apparently late-occurring lesions in mice and dogs; however, time course changes have not been systematically evaluated. Although mice were killed at intervals beginning at 13 weeks in one 2-year study, and hyperplastic lesions were induced in the urinary bladder, their incidences at different times were not presented (Schieferstein et al., 1985). Tumours in the urinary bladder are commonly not discovered until after about 2 years in mice (Schieferstein et al., 1985) and longer in dogs (Walpole et al., 1954; Deichmann et al., 1958, 1965). However, neoplastic transformation of human urothelial cells (infected with SV40) treated in vitro with 4-aminobiphenyl followed by in vitro culture for 6 weeks was demonstrated upon their inoculation into nude mice (Bookland et al., 1992b).

E. Strength, consistency, and specificity of association of the tumour response with key events

Evidence in support of the association of the tumour response with key events comes only in part from studies on bladder; considerable evidence is provided by studies on liver. DNA adduct formation has been demonstrated in both tissues.

There is an abundance of studies that demonstrate that 4-aminobiphenyl is a mutagen, including positive mutagenicity with certain frameshift mutation and base pair substitution-sensitive strains (TA1538, TA98, and TA100) of *Salmonella typhimurium*, but only in the presence of rodent liver S9 metabolic activating preparations. The requirement for S9 metabolic activation clearly demonstrates the lack of DNA reactivity and mutagenicity of the parent amine. In addition, 4-aminobiphenyl induces unscheduled DNA synthesis in rat liver cells in vitro (United States Environmental Protection Agency Genetic Activity Profiles). These in vitro studies provide evidence that 4-aminobiphenyl can cause genetic damage following metabolic activation. Bacterial mutation studies have also been conducted comparing metabolic activation systems based on liver homogenates from Aroclor 1254-induced male Sprague-Dawley rats and C57BL/6 mice, using *S. typhimurium* TA100 tester strains that expressed different levels of *N*- and *O*-acetyltransferase (OAT) activity (Dang & McQueen, 1999). TA100 has a single copy of the NAT/OAT gene; YG1029 has multiple copies of the NAT/OAT gene, and TA100/1,8DNP$_6$ is NAT/OAT-deficient. Effects with mouse and rat S9 were similar (but the effects of Aroclor 1254 treatment were not examined). Using either 4-aminobiphenyl or 4-acetylaminobiphenyl as substrates, considerably more mutations were induced in YG1029 than in TA100 or TA100/1,8DNP$_6$, in which mutation induction was similar. This supports a role for high acetylation activity in mutation induction by the *N*-hydroxylamine in these bacteria.

The non-enzymatic step to an arylnitrenium ion in the mechanism of mutagenesis in vivo is supported by the observation that *N*-hydroxy-4-aminobiphenyl mutagenesis in the high OAT-expressing *S. typhimurium* TG1024 strain is dependent on the pH of the medium, with an inverse relationship between mutant numbers and pH over the range 4.0–8.0 (Sarkar et al., 2002).

Administration of 4-aminobiphenyl in the drinking-water of BALB/c mice for 28 days resulted in higher levels of DNA adducts in liver than in urinary bladder of females, while the reverse occurred in males. Thus, in each sex, the DNA adduct level correlated with the susceptibility of the tissue to tumour induction by 4-aminobiphenyl (Poirier et al., 1995). However, the shape of the dose–response curve was linear for DNA adducts in both tissues (although it appears to saturate and is relatively flat in female mice), whereas the tumour dose–response curve was sigmoidal (Poirier et al., 1995).

Adduct levels were also highest in the urinary bladder of female Hsd:ICR(Br) mice that were dosed topically (the more usual exposure route in occupational settings) with 50 nmol 4-aminobiphenyl for 21 weeks. The principal adduct in all tissues examined (bladder, liver, lung, and skin) co-chromatographed with *N*-(deoxyguanosin-8-yl)-4-aminobiphenyl (Underwood et al., 1997).

One study of mutagenesis in male Muta™Mouse transgenic mice (i.e. transgenic CD2F, [BALB/c × DBA/2]) treated orally with 4-aminobiphenyl at 10 mg/kg bw per day for 10 days reported that the mutation frequencies in urinary bladder, liver, and bone marrow were increased by 13.7-, 4.8-, and 2.4-fold, respectively (Fletcher et al., 1998).

Newborn B6C3F1 (C57BL/6 × C3H) mice responded to treatment with 4-aminobiphenyl by developing a high frequency of liver tumours, many of which carried H-*ras* codon 61 CAA → AAA mutations (Parsons et al., 2005). In vivo, the level of one major DNA adduct [*N*-(deoxyguanosin-8-yl)-4-aminobiphenyl] was present at 5 adducts/10^6 nucleotides in newborn mice treated with 0.3 μmol 4-aminobiphenyl 24 h earlier. After 8 months, the CAA → AAA mutation was detected in 67% of the treated mice and 50% of the vehicle (dimethyl sulfoxide, or DMSO) controls, but the average mutant fraction in treated mice was 45×10^{-5} compared with only 2×10^{-5} in controls. After 12 months, liver tumours had developed in 79% of the treated mice and in 8% of the controls. These tumours are not those of the human target organ, but the results of this study support the general MOA proposed for bladder carcinogenesis (i.e. DNA adduct formation, followed by mutation in a key gene and the subsequent emergence of tumours).

Dogs (sex not stated) killed 24 h after a single oral dose of 4-aminobiphenyl (5 mg/kg bw) had 5.4 fmol DNA adducts/μg liver DNA and 4.8 fmol DNA adducts/μg urinary bladder DNA, whereas no DNA adducts were detected in either the liver or bladder of a dog whose bladder had been instilled with 4-aminobiphenyl. In contrast, a dog bladder instilled with the reactive intermediate *N*-hydroxy-4-aminobiphenyl had 3.9 fmol DNA adducts/μg bladder DNA and no detectable adducts in liver DNA. Quantification was by an immunochemical method (Roberts et al., 1988). Examination of bitches treated with tritium-labelled 4-aminobiphenyl (per os, intravenously, or intraurethrally), *N*-hydroxy-4-aminobiphenyl (intravenously or intraurethrally), or *N*-hydroxy-4-aminobiphenyl *N*-glucuronide (intravenously) demonstrated (1) the presence of 4-aminobiphenyl–haemoglobin adducts in blood erythrocytes; (2) that after per os dosing with 4-aminobiphenyl, the major portion of total *N*-hydroxy-4-aminobiphenyl entering the bladder lumen was free *N*-hydroxy-4-aminobiphenyl (0.7%), with lower concentrations of the acid-labile *N*-glucuronide (0.3%); (3) that urothelial DNA adducts following intraurethral instillation of *N*-hydroxy-4-aminobiphenyl were 60 times higher than after intraurethral instillation of 4-aminobiphenyl; and (4) that exposure to *N*-hydroxy-4-aminobiphenyl and subsequent 4-aminobiphenyl–DNA adduct formation are directly dependent on the frequency of urination and, to a lesser extent, on urinary pH (Kadlubar et al., 1991). The urinary pH of dogs may vary from about 4.5 to 7.5, depending upon the diet (Merck, 1998), time after eating, time of day, and amount of water consumed; these are factors that might influence the carcinogenic response (Cohen, 1995). Studies in vitro with microsomal preparations from dog liver and bladder have shown the presence of transacetylation activities in both organs, so that *N*-hydroxy-4-aminobiphenyl binding to RNA and DNA occurs in the presence of 4-acetylaminobiphenyl, *N*-hydroxy-4-acetyl-aminobiphenyl, or acetyl coenzyme A (CoA) as acetyl donors, although the levels of binding were less with bladder than with hepatic microsomes (Hatcher & Swaminathan, 1992).

Examination of urothelial cells exfoliated into urine of dogs treated with 4-aminobiphenyl showed that DNA adducts were identical to those from DNA modified in vitro with *N*-hydroxy-4-aminobiphenyl and from dog bladder urothelial DNA isolated from 4-amino-biphenyl-dosed dogs at autopsy. A dose-related increase in 4-aminobiphenyl–DNA adduct formation was demonstrated (Talaska et al., 1990).

F. Biological plausibility and coherence

The observations that 4-aminobiphenyl can form adducts with DNA and that it is mutagenic in organs in which tumours develop indicate, in general terms, that the proposed MOA is plausible (Fletcher et al., 1998). In addition, *N*-hydroxy-4-aminobiphenyl is able to cause neoplastic transformation of non-tumorigenic SV40-immortalized human urothelial cells (Bookland et al., 1992b). The findings with 4-aminobiphenyl are also consistent with the vast literature regarding the metabolic activation, DNA adduct formation, mutagenesis, and urinary bladder carcinogenesis in several species (including humans) of several related aromatic amine chemicals (Kadlubar et al., 1977; Miller & Miller, 1977; Delclos et al., 1987). The lack of DNA adduct formation and mutagenicity of the parent amine in various in vitro systems without metabolic activation clearly demonstrates the requirement for metabolic activation. The same DNA adducts are identified in tissues after administration of the amine or following exposure to the *N*-hydroxyl metabolite, with the structure of the adducts having been chemically confirmed. The mutagenic potential of the specific C-8 guanine DNA adduct has also been demonstrated, although the specific biophysical aspects have been better demonstrated for structurally related aromatic amines such as 2-aminofluorene (Kriek, 1992).

G. Other modes of action

Alternatives of components of the already described MOA have been suggested. However, they do not detract from the overall described MOA but suggest either alternative specific aspects (such as other activating enzymes) or associative processes that could affect quantitative aspects. 4-Aminobiphenyl is oxidized by hepatic enzymes other than CYP1A2 (Kimura et al., 1999) to the *N*-hydroxylated metabolite that causes liver and urinary bladder toxicity and carcinogenesis, possibly including oxidases and peroxidases (Kadlubar et al., 1982, 1991). Although the specific enzymes involved in metabolic activation may vary, the ultimate sequence of generation of a reactive electrophile, DNA adduct formation, mutagenesis, and carcinogenesis is consistent. Furthermore, it is reasonable to believe that from this point in the MOA, the same sequence occurs as that involving CYP1A2-mediated activation, regardless of the activating enzyme.

In addition to bulky adducts, there is evidence to suggest that *N*-hydroxy-4-aminobiphenyl causes oxidative damage in urothelial DNA, possibly involving endogenous peroxidases (Burger et al., 2001). The relevance of this for the carcinogenic activity of 4-aminobiphenyl is unknown.

N-Hydroxy-4-aminobiphenyl and its further activated forms are cytotoxic to urothelial and other cells in vitro (Reznikoff et al., 1986), but the role that this plays in its carcinogenic effects is unclear (see below for discussion of a potentiating role in urothelial carcinogenesis, rather than causative role). It is likely that this process alters the dose–response relationship, but does not alter the fundamental MOA described above.

H. Assessment of the postulated mode of action

The early steps in the proposed MOA are well supported by the available evidence, and it has been judged that there is good and sufficient evidence that 4-aminobiphenyl is a urinary bladder carcinogen in dogs and mice, and in other tissues (primarily the liver) in rodents. Thus, it is metabolized to products that can form DNA adducts in the liver and in other target organs, and mutations have been demonstrated to arise. Although other organs can also be targets for 4-aminobiphenyl-induced neoplasia, the urinary bladder is the main target in dogs and in some strains of mice. Evidence for the intervening steps between general genotoxicity and the emergence of neoplasia is lacking. There is a notable lack of study of the effects of 4-aminobiphenyl on cell proliferation in the urinary bladder, but information on related aromatic amines and amides is available, particularly the analysis of the interaction between DNA reactivity (and mutagenesis) and cell proliferation induced by 2-acetylaminofluorene in mouse urinary bladder utilizing data from a megamouse, ED-01 study (Cairns, 1979; Gaylor, 1979; Littlefield et al., 1979). The reliance for mutagenicity on cell proliferation can provide an explanation for the sigmoidal shape of the tumour dose–response despite a linear dose–response for DNA adducts (Cohen & Ellwein, 1990). This link has significant implications for assessing potency and dose–response for 4-aminobiphenyl-induced urinary bladder cancer (see discussion below).

I. Uncertainties, inconsistencies, and data gaps

Bacterial mutation studies of 4-aminobiphenyl with metabolic activation have shown that most mutations are frameshifts, whereas a single study of sequence analysis of 4-aminobiphenyl-induced mutations in the *lacZ* gene in single-stranded DNA from a bacteriophage M13 cloning vector revealed exclusively base pair substitutions, with over 80% occurring at G sites: G → T transversions predominated, followed by G → C transversions and G → A transitions. The major DNA adduct, *N*-(deoxyguanosin-8-yl)-4-aminobiphenyl, was then inserted within the M13 genome, and the mutational frequency and specificity were measured after in vivo replication. The targeted mutational efficiency was approximately 0.01%, and the primary mutation was G → C transversion. Thus, the observations are consistent with in vivo observations, but the mutagenic activity was weak (Verghis et al., 1997).

Most in vivo investigations have been in mice. Dogs, for understandable reasons, have received less attention, although this is the species that is more sensitive to bladder carcinogenesis. Mouse strain differences in response are evident: B6C3F1 and female BALB/cStCrlfC3Hf/Nctr are more susceptible to liver carcinogenesis, whereas male BALB/cStCrlfC3Hf/Nctr mice develop bladder tumours after exposure to 4-aminobiphenyl (Schieferstein et al., 1985; Dooley et al., 1988, 1992). Nevertheless, mouse strain effects have received relatively little attention in the available studies.

The enzyme considered as fundamental for the metabolism of 4-aminobiphenyl to a product that forms adducts with DNA in liver and bladder is CYP1A2 (Butler et al., 1989a, 1989b). However, comparison of responses in CYP1A2(+/+) wild-type mice with CYP1A2(−/−) knockout mice showed that, contrary to expectations, CYP1A2 expression was not associated with 4-aminobiphenyl-induced oxidative stress or with 4-aminobiphenyl–DNA adduct formation. Furthermore, prior treatment with 2,3,7,8-tetrachlorodibenzo-*p*-dioxin (TCDD), which increased hepatic CYP1A2 protein expression 5-fold along with expression of other phase I and phase II enzymes, either did not change or actually decreased the level of adducts in liver. The specific quantitative effects of such induction will depend on the balance of the enzymes induced. These results suggest either that CYP1A2 is not the major metabolic activator of 4-aminobiphenyl or that other enzymes in mice activate the compound in the absence of CYP1A2 (Tsuneoka et al., 2003). Based on studies with other aromatic amines, additional activating enzymes might include other P-450 enzymes, oxidases, or peroxidases (Lakshmi et al., 1990; Smith et al., 1991; Hughes et al., 1992).

Another reaction considered to be important for carcinogenesis induced by 4-aminobiphenyl is acetylation. Acetylation plays several roles in 4-aminobiphenyl carcinogenesis. *O*-Acetylation and *N,O*-acetyltransfer of *N*-hydroxy-4-aminobiphenyl are expected to increase risk in humans, whereas *N*-acetylation of 4-aminobiphenyl should reduce risk (Lower et al., 1979). Acetylation can be catalysed by NAT1 or NAT2, with the latter exhibiting a marked polymorphism within the population (Hein et al., 2000; Cascorbi et al., 2001). It is predicted that a slow acetylation phenotype will increase the risk of bladder cancer, since acetylation of the parent amine, 4-aminobiphenyl, is considered to be a detoxification process in humans, whereas a rapid acetylation phenotype should be associated with a decreased risk.

However, studies of acetylator phenotype in mice have produced conflicting results. In one study, male and female homozygous rapid acetylator or homozygous slow acetylator mice that were apparently identical in every other respect were administered 4-aminobiphenyl·HCl (55–300 mg/l) in drinking-water for 28 days. The levels of hepatic DNA adducts increased with dose in both sexes, with the levels being higher in females, but were independent of the mouse acetylator phenotype. In the urinary bladder, DNA adducts increased to a plateau at 100 mg/kg in male mice and were again independent of acetylator phenotype. In female mice, the DNA adduct levels were lower than in males and decreased at the highest dose; the DNA adduct levels were higher in the rapid acetylator phenotype, contrary to expectations (Flammang et al., 1992). These results were interpreted as suggesting that acetyltransferase activities are not rate determining for DNA adduct formation in mice. A similar conclusion that there was no correlation between murine *NAT2* alleles and 4-aminobiphenyl–DNA adduct levels was reached by McQueen et al. (2003), using C57BL/6, B6.A, and A/J mouse strains and the transgenic strains hNAT1:A/J and hNAT1:C57, which carry the human *NAT1* transgene. However, the differences in murine NAT2 activity were modest and probably not sufficient to affect 4-aminobiphenyl genotoxicity. Recent studies suggest that in humans, NAT1, not NAT2, is responsible for the *O*-acetylation of *N*-hydroxy-4-aminobiphenyl (Oda, 2004).

There are also mouse strain-specific mutations that require explanation. Thus, in B6C3F1, 4-aminobiphenyl induces predominantly C $\rightarrow$ A mutations (reflecting G $\rightarrow$ T transversions in the non-coding strand) in H-*ras* codon 61, whereas in CD-1 mice, the predominant mutation in H-*ras* codon 61 was A $\rightarrow$ T transversion (Manjanatha et al., 1996).

Cell proliferation is also required for neoplasia, but there have been few studies that have investigated cell proliferation at an early stage of the carcinogenic process of 4-aminobiphenyl. It is also notable that in the carcinogenicity experiment described previously (Schieferstein et al., 1985), although urinary bladder carcinomas developed only in males, a high prevalence of hyperplasia was reported in both males and females. Apparently this observation has not been investigated further (discussed below).

In summary, the evidence is strong for the sequence of key events including metabolic activation, DNA adduct formation, and gene mutation as the MOA for 4-aminobiphenyl-induced urinary bladder carcinogenesis. It is further strengthened by data from studies with structurally related aromatic amines. However, data gaps remain concerning details of the specific enzymes involved, the basis for differing organ specificity between species and details regarding potency, and the shape of the dose–response curve in humans. This is, perhaps, not unexpected in view of the complexity of the relevant competing metabolic pathways. While available data are considered sufficient to support the hypothesized MOA, the impact of these uncertainties needs to be considered quantitatively in the overall assessment (Table 3).

Table 3. Modulating factors affecting 4-aminobiphenyl urinary bladder carcinogenesis.

1.	Competing activities of esterification enzymes
2.	Genetic polymorphisms affecting enzymatic activation or inactivation (e.g. slow and fast acetylators)
3.	Urinary pH (mainly affected by diet) and possibly other urinary constituents
4.	Urothelial cell proliferation (induced by high doses of 4-aminobiphenyl or by co-administration with some other agent affecting urothelial proliferation)

CAN HUMAN RELEVANCE OF THE MOA BE REASONABLY EXCLUDED ON THE BASIS OF FUNDAMENTAL, QUALITATIVE DIFFERENCES IN KEY EVENTS BETWEEN EXPERIMENTAL ANIMALS AND HUMANS?

There is considerable evidence in humans and human cell systems supporting each of the key events for 4-aminobiphenyl-induced urinary bladder cancer. Metabolic activation to the *N*-hydroxylamine has been demonstrated, with several different enzymes being suggested for activation and several others that might potentiate or reduce the effects of *N*-hydroxylation, such as *N*-acetylation. Genetic polymorphisms significantly affect activities of these enzymes, producing variations in the population that can affect susceptibility to the urinary bladder carcinogenesis response to 4-aminobiphenyl exposures. DNA adducts identical to those detected in DNA from mice and dogs have been identified in human urothelial cells, and consequently they have a similar mutagenic potential. Furthermore, extensive epidemiological evidence demonstrates the urinary bladder carcinogenicity of 4-aminobiphenyl in humans.

Bladder cancer is associated with smoking and occupational exposures to 4-aminobiphenyl. 4-Aminobiphenyl was manufactured in the United States of America from 1935 to 1955 (Melick et al., 1955) and was used as a highly efficient rubber antioxidant, but it is apparently no longer commercially produced. In epidemiological studies, which were confined to one series of workers occupationally exposed to commercial 4-aminobiphenyl, a high incidence of bladder carcinomas was reported (Melick et al., 1955, 1971; Melamed et al., 1960; Koss et al., 1965, 1969). Among 503 workers, 59 cases with positive cytology were identified, among which 35 cases of carcinoma of the urinary bladder were histologically verified; 7 remained cytologically positive at the time of publication, while 7 died from other causes and 10 were lost to follow-up (Koss et al., 1969). In addition to cigarette smoke, there also appear to be other, ill-defined environmental sources of exposure, possibly from other sources of combustion of substances containing carbon and nitrogen (Skipper et al., 2003). Cigarette

56

smoking accounts for between 40% and 70% of the bladder cancer cases in the United States and Europe (IARC, 1986; Castelao et al., 2001). Black (air-cured) tobacco is a greater source of 4-aminobiphenyl than is blonde (flue-cured) tobacco (Bryant et al., 1988).

The key events demonstrated for 4-aminobiphenyl bladder carcinogenesis in mice and dogs have also been specifically evaluated for 4-aminobiphenyl in humans, primarily in individuals exposed to 4-aminobiphenyl in cigarette smoke, but also utilizing in vitro methods with human urothelial cells (see Table 4).

Table 4. Concordance evaluation of key events of 4-aminobiphenyl-induced urinary bladder carcinogenesis between species.

Key event	Mouse	Dog	Human
1. Metabolic activation to reactive electrophile	+	+	+
2. DNA adduct formation	+	+	+
3. Mutagenesis	+	+	+
4. Carcinoma	+	+	+

Absorbed 4-aminobiphenyl is N-oxidized in the liver by CYP1A2, which, in spite of its rather high homology with CYP1A1, has an essentially different substrate specificity and is found only in liver (Lang & Pelkonen, 1999). Other enzymes have been suggested to be capable of supporting metabolic activation to the N-hydroxylamine.

NAT1 and NAT2 each catalyse three types of acetylation: the N-acetylation of arylamines, the O-acetylation of N-hydroxylamines, and the N,O-acetyltransfer of arylhydroxamic acids (Flammang & Kadlubar, 1986; Mattano et al., 1989; Fretland et al., 1997; Hein et al., 2000). It is believed that N-acetylation by N-acetyltransferases has a protective effect regarding bladder carcinogenicity, primarily because the acetamide of 4-aminobiphenyl formed is significantly less potent as a substrate for N-hydroxylation compared with the amine. Two genes, *NAT1* and *NAT2*, code for the NAT isoforms, and allelic variation has been associated with susceptibility to urinary bladder cancer in humans (Hein et al., 2000). Most studies suggest that NAT2 slow acetylators are at increased risk of developing bladder cancer, whereas the contribution of the *NAT1* genotype to aromatic amine bladder carcinogenesis is less clear (Cartwright et al., 1982; Hein et al., 2000). Among smokers, there is a higher level of 4-aminobiphenyl–haemoglobin adducts associated with the slow acetylator phenotype (Vineis et al., 1990). Interactions of *NAT1* and *NAT2* have been suggested (Cascorbi et al., 2001). In a study of 425 German bladder cancer patients, Cascorbi et al. (2001) found that there is (1) a partial linkage of the *NAT1*10* genotype to the *NAT2*4* genotype, (2) a clear underrepresentation of *NAT1*10* genotypes among rapid *NAT2* genotypes in the cases studied, and (3) a gene–gene–environment interaction in that *NAT2*slow/NAT1*4* genotype combinations with a history of occupational exposure were 5.96 (2.96–12.0) times more frequent in cancer cases than in controls without a risk from occupation ($P < 0.0001$). Hence, the data suggest that individuals with *NAT2*4* and *NAT1*10* are at a significantly lower risk for bladder cancer, particularly when exposed to environmental risk factors.

Polymorphisms in *CYP1A2* (Oscarson et al., n.d.) and *NAT2* (Hein et al., 2000) genes are associated with variations in the activities of these enzymes in human populations, although the extent to which variation in CYP1A2 activity is due to genetic factors has yet to be determined (Sachse et al., 2003). Moreover, expression of the *CYP1A2* gene is induced in cigarette smokers, leading to even higher CYP1A2 enzyme activities (Sesardic et al., 1988; Eaton et al., 1995). An individual exposed to 4-aminobiphenyl and expressing high levels of CYP1A2 and slow NAT2 activity would be expected to have increased levels of *N*-hydroxy-4-aminobiphenyl and, therefore, higher levels of 4-aminobiphenyl–haemoglobin adducts and 4-aminobiphenyl–DNA adducts in liver and urinary bladder than an individual expressing low levels of CYP1A2 and rapid NAT2 activity.

The tumour suppressor genes *RB1* and *TP53* appear to be involved in bladder cancer, especially high-grade urothelial carcinomas rather than low-grade papillary tumours. Both genes are involved in the regulation of the cell cycle. In addition, *TP53* plays a role in response to DNA damage, cell death, and neovascularization (Hickman et al., 2002), and its gene product regulates the expression of multiple genes (Vousden & Lu, 2002). A strong association has been found between *RB1* inactivation and muscle invasion (Cairns et al., 1991; Ishikawa et al., 1991; Presti et al., 1991; Primdahl et al., 2000). In one study of 45 bladder cancers, seven of nine *TP53* mutations occurred in grade 3 tumours (i.e. invasion includes perivesicular tissue) (Martone et al., 1998). Inactivation of *RB1* occurs in 30–80% of muscle-invasive bladder cancers (Cairns et al., 1991; Logothetis et al., 1992; Wright et al., 1995; Ioachim et al., 2000), most frequently as a consequence of heterozygous 13q deletions in combination with mutation of the remaining allele (Cordon-Cardo & Reuter, 1997). In studies investigating at least 30 tumours, *TP53* mutations occurred in 40–60% of invasive bladder cancers (Tiguert et al., 2001; Lu et al., 2002). Although no specific mutational hotspots were identified, more than 90% of the mutations occurred in exons 4–9. In a study of the binding spectrum of *N*-hydroxy-4-aminobiphenyl in DNA fragments containing exons 5, 7, and 8 of *TP53*, preferential binding was identified at codon 285, a non-CpG site, and at codons 175 and 248, which are CpG sites, but only after C5 cytosine methylation had occurred (Feng et al., 2002). The authors concluded that the mutational spectrum in *TP53* in bladder cancer strongly suggests a role of 4-aminobiphenyl in the etiology of this neoplasm.

Exposure to tobacco smoke, an environmental source of 4-aminobiphenyl, is associated with increased levels of 4-aminobiphenyl–haemoglobin adducts, in both adults and fetuses. In a study of smoking ($n = 14$) and non-smoking ($n = 38$) women, 4-aminobiphenyl–haemoglobin levels were 183 ± 108 pg/g haemoglobin in smokers and 22 ± 8 pg/g haemoglobin in non-smokers, whereas the levels in their respective fetuses were 92 ± 54 pg/g haemoglobin and 17 ± 13 pg/g haemoglobin (Coghlin et al., 1991), a difference that has also been observed in adults in studies of tumour tissue DNA (Curigliano et al., 1996). Haemoglobin adduct levels (used as a surrogate for exposure levels and indicator for DNA adduct potential) have been associated with levels of exposure to tobacco as a source of 4-aminobiphenyl (black tobacco > blonde tobacco > non-smokers) in a male study population from Turin, Italy; the risk of bladder cancer followed the same pattern (Bryant et al., 1988). There is a substantial gap in information linking the presence of adducts, primarily an indication of exposure, and the emergence of cancer.

In humans, 4-aminobiphenyl has been associated only with urinary bladder cancer, whereas in mice, liver and urinary bladder tumours are induced. Although the specific reasons for these species differences in organ specificity are not known, they appear to be due to variations in competing *N*-esterification enzymatic activations. Sulfation appears to be primarily associated with liver carcinogenesis by aromatic amines, whereas *N*-glucuronidation appears to be more associated with bladder carcinogenesis. Acetylation has mixed effects, but in humans appears to be principally a detoxification process that can be influenced significantly by *N*-acetyltransferase polymorphisms that result in fast versus slow acetylation. Human tissues have been studied for their possible involvement in the metabolism of 4-aminobiphenyl and its metabolites. CYP1A2 is responsible for the metabolism of 4-aminobiphenyl to *N*-hydroxy-4-aminobiphenyl by human hepatic microsomal fraction (Butler et al., 1989b). *N*-Hydroxy-4-aminobiphenyl can be metabolized to a product that binds covalently to calf thymus DNA by cytosolic sulfotransferases from human liver and, to a lesser extent, colon, but not from pancreas or urinary bladder. In view of this lack of sulfotransferase activity in bladder, it has been suggested that hepatic sulfotransferase may actually decrease the bioavailability of *N*-hydroxy-4-aminobiphenyl in extrahepatic tissues and serve as a detoxification mechanism for the urinary bladder (Chou et al., 1995). On the other hand, *N*-acetyltransferases that are present in human urothelial cells (Frederickson et al., 1992; Swaminathan & Reznikoff, 1992) can metabolize *N*-hydroxy-4-aminobiphenyl, as well as the acetylated compounds *N*-hydroxy-4-acetylaminobiphenyl and *N*-acetoxy-4-acetylaminobiphenyl, to a DNA-reactive material. The major adduct co-chromatographs with *N*-(deoxyguanosin-8-yl)-4-aminobiphenyl. ^{32}P-postlabelling analysis of the DNA from cytosol-mediated binding of *N*-hydroxy-4-aminobiphenyl revealed four radioactive spots. Five adducts were found when intact human urothelial cells were used, two of which were the same as two found using cytosol. This suggests the possibility of an activation pathway or pathways in addition to acetylation.

Experiments similar to those performed with dog tissues have shown that human urothelial cell microsomes possess transacetylation activity, so that *N*-hydroxy-4-aminobiphenyl binding to RNA and DNA occurs in the presence of 4-acetylaminobiphenyl, *N*-hydroxy-4-acetylaminobiphenyl, or acetylCoA as acetyl donors (Hatcher et al., 1993). These authors also found that ^{32}P-postlabelling of DNA adducts formed after reaction with *N*-hydroxy-4-aminobiphenyl, *N*-hydroxy-4-acetylaminobiphenyl, and *N*-acetoxy-4-aminobiphenyl showed similar profiles, suggesting that the arylnitrenium ion, arising from *N*-acetoxy-4-aminobiphenyl, might be the common reactive species. The structures of the adducts have been identified as the 3′,5′-bisphospho derivatives of *N*-(deoxyguanosin-8-yl)-4-aminobiphenyl (dG-C8-aminobiphenyl), *N*-(deoxyadenosin-8-yl)-4-aminobiphenyl (dA-C8-aminobiphenyl) (Frederickson et al., 1992; Hatcher & Swaminathan, 1995), and *N*-(deoxyguanosin-*N*(2)-yl)-4-azobiphenyl (Hatcher & Swaminathan, 2002).

The results available comparing tobacco smokers with non-smokers support the relevance to humans of the hypothesized MOA. In a study of 46 T1 bladder cancer cases, mean relative staining intensity for 4-aminobiphenyl–DNA adducts was significantly higher in current smokers (275 ± 81, $n = 24$) than in non-smokers (113 ± 71, $n = 22$) (Curigliano et al., 1996). Similar results have been reported for laryngeal tissue (Flamini et al., 1998) and for mammary tissue (Faraglia et al., 2003). Using 4-aminobiphenyl–haemoglobin adducts as an indicator of exposure, it was found that bladder carcinoma patients had higher levels than controls (Del Santo et al., 1991), whereas lung cancer patients did not (Weston et al., 1991). The basis for this difference is unknown.

In addition to the evidence of genotoxicity generated with non-human test systems, 4-amino-biphenyl can be metabolized by human urothelial cell microsomal preparations to a mutagen in *S. typhimurium* YG1024 (a derivative of TA98 with elevated *O*-acetyltransferase activity) but not in strain TA98 itself (Hatcher et al., 1993). No other species or other human tissues were examined in this study.

6-Thioguanine-resistant mutants can be induced in a non-tumorigenic, SV40-immortalized human urothelial cell line by exposure to 4-aminobiphenyl itself or exposure to *N*-hydroxy-4-aminobiphenyl, *N*-hydroxy-4-acetylaminobiphenyl, or *N*-acetoxy-4-acetylaminobiphenyl (Bookland et al., 1992a). No exogenous metabolic activation system was required for the observed activity. The lowest effective concentrations to produce a statistically significant increase in the mutant fraction were as follows: *N*-acetoxy-4-acetylaminobiphenyl, 2 µmol/l; *N*-hydroxy-4-acetylaminobiphenyl, 5 µmol/l; *N*-hydroxy-4-aminobiphenyl, 20 µmol/l; and 4-aminobiphenyl, 100 µmol/l. Three of these substances were also tested for tumorigenic transformation using the same human immortalized urothelial cells in an in vitro–in vivo assay in which the end-point was carcinoma development when treated cells were injected subcutaneously into nude mice (Bookland et al., 1992b). Transformation was demonstrated after all treatments, the lowest concentrations being as follows: *N*-hydroxy-4-acetylamino-biphenyl, 0.5 µmol/l; *N*-hydroxy-4-aminobiphenyl, 0.5 µmol/l; and 4-aminobiphenyl, 20 µmol/l. The lower concentrations required for transformation in comparison with those for mutation are noted, but how this should be interpreted is not clear. It is consistent with the transformation being independent of mutation and with the transformation assay having a higher sensitivity, or it could merely reflect a difference in sensitivity of the methods.

In summary, on a qualitative basis, the key events in the MOA are the same in mice, dogs, and humans: metabolic activation to the *N*-hydroxylamine with subsequent formation of a reactive electrophile (presumably the nitrenium ion), formation of guanine adducts, gene mutation, and the ultimate formation of cancer. The intervening events between gene mutation and cancer, such as which genes are mutated and how cancer is induced, are not known. The MOA, nevertheless, has been clearly demonstrated and is the same in the animal models and in humans.

CAN HUMAN RELEVANCE OF THE MOA BE REASONABLY EXCLUDED ON THE BASIS OF QUANTITATIVE DIFFERENCES IN EITHER KINETIC OR DYNAMIC FACTORS BETWEEN EXPERIMENTAL ANIMALS AND HUMANS?

As described in detail above, the metabolic activation, DNA adducts, and mutagenicity of 4-aminobiphenyl are qualitatively the same in mice, dogs, and humans, leading to the induction of urothelial tumours of the urinary bladder in these three species and other tumours in mice, rats, and rabbits. Although detailed aspects of absorption, distribution, and excretion have not been reported, similarity in the levels of DNA adduct formation in the urothelium occurring in mice, dogs, and humans suggests that kinetic differences are not significant between these three species. Although similar enzymatic processes occur in the three species, quantitative differences are evident. These differences may explain some of the variations seen in target organ specificity among the species and might suggest possible quantitative differences in generation of the DNA adducts. Nevertheless, these differences do not negate the overall MOA for any of the species or the different target organs and are consistent with the complexity of the competing pathways for metabolic activation and deactivation.

Presumably there is a potential for repair of the different adducts, and quantitative differences might exist among species and even among tissues. However, the detection of relatively high numbers of adducts in all three species indicates that significant numbers of stable adducts are produced.

The target tissue common among mice, dogs, and humans, the urinary bladder urothelium, is similar morphologically (Pauli et al., 1983). The urothelium has a characteristic asymmetric unit membrane at the luminal surface that provides a major part of the barrier function to urine. It is composed of urothelium-specific proteins, the uroplakins, the sequence of which is highly conserved among species (Wu et al., 1994). In addition, the urothelium is metabolically active in all three species.

Modulating urinary factors have also been identified that can quantitatively affect the ultimate formation of urothelial DNA adducts, such as pH and frequency of urination (Cohen, 1995; Sarkar et al., 2002). Although the range of pH varies among species, the pH in mice, dogs, and humans readily reaches acidic and alkaline levels as well as neutral. Again, although quantitative differences occur, these do not preclude the existence of this MOA in humans.

There is no evidence implicating another MOA besides DNA reactivity. However, significant quantitative differences exist between species with regard to apparent potency of 4-aminobiphenyl with respect to urinary bladder carcinogenesis. It is clear, however, that metabolites of 4-aminobiphenyl interact with proteins (e.g. haemoglobin) as well as with DNA and that metabolites of 4-aminobiphenyl are cytotoxic (Schieferstein et al., 1985; Reznikoff et al., 1986; Kadlubar et al., 1991). Interaction with urothelial cellular proteins might be responsible for the cytotoxicity and regenerative proliferation seen in the mouse bladder at higher doses of 4-aminobiphenyl. The interaction of DNA reactivity and consequent mutagenicity and cell proliferation provide an explanation for the sigmoidal shape of the dose–response curve for tumours despite a linear dose–response for DNA adducts (Cohen & Ellwein, 1990). The high concentrations of 4-aminobiphenyl found in the urine of mice that can produce urothelial cytotoxicity are generally not attained in humans exposed to cigarette smoke. However, other (unknown) substances appear to produce urothelial hyperplasia in cigarette smokers (Auerbach & Garfinkel, 1989). This increased cell proliferation significantly potentiates the effects of 4-aminobiphenyl on the bladder, providing a significantly greater number of DNA-replicating cell targets on which to act in comparison with the small number present in the normal, slowly replicating urothelium. Thus, the apparent greater potency of 4-aminobiphenyl in humans compared with mice is unlikely, but represents the synergy of DNA reactivity and cell proliferation produced by a single substance, 4-aminobiphenyl, in mice, but by different substances in the complex mixture of cigarette smoke.

Occupational exposure to 4-aminobiphenyl presumably resulted in greater doses of 4-amino-biphenyl than did exposure to cigarette smoke, since the incidence of bladder cancer in such populations was considerably higher than in smokers. However, quantitative measurements of metabolite concentrations or DNA adduct levels in urothelial cells could not be determined at the time these occupational exposures occurred, and cigarette smoking history in those individuals was not assessed (Koss et al., 1965, 1969).

In summary, although quantitative differences among species exist, they do not exclude the same MOA in mice and dogs occurring in humans.

CONCLUSION: STATEMENT OF CONFIDENCE, ANALYSIS, AND IMPLICATIONS

The early steps in the proposed MOA are well supported by the available evidence, indicating that the key events of metabolic activation, DNA adduct formation, and mutation are the same qualitatively in mice, dogs, and humans. There is strong and sufficient evidence that 4-aminobiphenyl is a human urinary bladder carcinogen. Evidence for the intervening steps between mutation and cancer development is lacking. The associations described for adduct levels and *TP53* mutations are not compelling because these particular genetic alterations appear late in tumour progression and are often the result of endogenous causes (e.g. spontaneous depurination at methylated CpG sites). This aspect of *TP53* mutations in bladder cancer has been studied in a case–control study (Schroeder et al., 2003). In addition, most urothelial tumours in humans are low-grade papillary lesions, which generally do not have *TP53* mutations.

The mutational spectrum of *N*-hydroxy-4-acetylaminobiphenyl has been studied in embryonic fibroblasts of the Big Blue mouse (Besaratinia et al., 2002). Treatment of these cells for 24 h resulted in a dose-dependent increase in mutation frequency of the *cII* transgene of up to 12.8-fold over background. Single-base substitutions comprised 86% of the mutations in the treated cells and 74% of the mutations in the controls. Of these mutations, 63% and 36%, respectively, occurred at guanine residues along the *cII* gene. Whereas G → T transversions accounted for 47% of the mutations in the treated *cII* gene, the most common mutations in untreated cells were insertions, which accounted for 19% of the mutations. Mapping of the induced adducts established five preferred DNA adduction sites, of which four were major mutation sites for *N*-hydroxy-4-acetoxyaminobiphenyl, especially G → T transversions. In the *TP53* gene in human bladder cancer, however, G → A transitions predominate (53%) and are prevalent at all of its five mutational hotspots (codons 175, 248, 273, 280, and 285), three of which are at methylated CpG hotspots (175, 248, and 273). In *cII*, neither the preferred adduction sites nor the induced mutational hotspots are biased towards methylated CpG dinucleotides. It is concluded from this study that there is a serious discordance between the mutation pattern induced by *N*-hydroxy-4-acetoxyaminobiphenyl in the *cII* gene and the mutational pattern observed in *TP53* in human bladder cancer. However, the role of methylation status and transcriptional activity on the mutation spectrum induced by 4-aminobiphenyl has yet to be determined. It is also to be noted that the *TP53* mutation spectrum is a reflection of a selection process during tumour development.

Based on the preceding analysis, it is clear that the MOA for 4-aminobiphenyl carcinogenesis is known in the animal model, and the MOA is relevant to humans both qualitatively and quantitatively. The conclusion based on this evaluation, even without epidemiological evidence, is that 4-aminobiphenyl poses a cancer hazard to humans.

To perform a full risk assessment requires additional information regarding the dose–response and human exposures. Based on the information described above, it is clear that the data predict a cancer hazard for humans at expected exposures, at least for occupational (historical) and cigarette smoking exposures. Further analysis is required regarding the potential risk at ambient exposures in those who are not cigarette smokers. The MOA analysis provides the basis and foundation for such an assessment. The epidemiological evidence on 4-aminobiphenyl supports the conclusions suggested by the MOA HRF.

4-AMINOBIPHENYL AND THE HUMAN RELEVANCE FRAMEWORK

4-Aminobiphenyl was evaluated using the proposed IPCS HRF based on an MOA analysis. The defined key events for this DNA reactivity MOA—metabolic activation, DNA adduct formation, mutagenicity, and cancer induction—clearly are the same in humans as in the animal (mice, dogs) models, indicating that 4-aminobiphenyl presents a cancer hazard for humans. The information for this MOA analysis provides a substantive foundation on which to build a complete cancer risk assessment for humans. For this chemical, there is also substantial epidemiological evidence to verify the conclusions derived from the HRF analysis.

The additional key events for this MOA—which genes are mutated and how do these genetic alterations lead to cancer—are not known for 4-aminobiphenyl. However, this does not detract from the conclusions, given the strength of evidence for the proposed MOA, based on the framework analysis presented here.

What data are necessary to conclude that a chemical produces cancer by a DNA-reactive MOA? Our suggestion is that at the very least there be a demonstration that DNA adducts are produced, preferably in the target tissue, and that the chemical is mutagenic (either with or without metabolic activation). Mutagenicity is used here in a more specific, restricted sense than the broader term genotoxicity. Demonstration of DNA adducts and mutagenicity in the target tissue after in vivo exposure increases confidence in the proposed MOA. Identification of the specific metabolic pathway and specific DNA adducts induced provides a significantly better basis for extrapolating between the animal model and humans.

This case demonstrates the potential utility of data on surrogate compounds in MOA analysis. However, the relevance of data on related compounds, whether in vivo or in vitro, needs to be adequately justified. Weight-of-evidence analysis of structure–activity relationships, which have been well developed for DNA reactivity and mutagenicity, should also contribute to framework analysis.

ACKNOWLEDGEMENTS

This paper has been reviewed in accordance with United States Environmental Protection Agency (USEPA) guidance but does not necessarily reflect USEPA policy. We thank Drs. Andrew Kligerman and Doug Wolf for their careful review of this paper.

REFERENCES

al-Atrash J, Zhang YJ, Lin D, Kadlubar FF, Santella RM (1995) Quantitative immunohistochemical analysis of 4-aminobiphenyl–DNA cultured cells and mice: Comparison to gas chromatography/mass spectroscopy analysis. *Chemical Research in Toxicology*, **8**:747–752.

Auerbach O, Garfinkel L (1989) Histologic changes in the urinary bladder in relation to cigarette smoking and use of artificial sweeteners. *Cancer*, **64**:983–987.

Besaratinia A, Bates SE, Pfeifer GP (2002) Mutational signature of the proximate bladder carcinogen *N*-hydroxy-4-acetylaminobiphenyl: Inconsistency with the *p53* mutational spectrum in bladder cancer. *Cancer Research*, **62**:4331–4338.

Block NL, Sigel MM, Lynne CM, Ng AB, Grosberg RA (1978) The initiation, progress, and diagnosis of dog bladder cancer induced by 4-aminobiphenyl. *Investigative Urology*, **16**:50–54.

Bonser GM (1962) Precancerous changes in the urinary bladder. In: Severi L, ed. *The morphological precursor of cancer*. Perugia, University of Perugia, p. 435.

Bookland EA, Reznikoff CA, Lindstrom M, Swaminathan S (1992a) Induction of thioguanine-resistant mutations in human uroepithelial cells by 4-aminobiphenyl and its *N*-hydroxy derivatives. *Cancer Research*, **52**:1615–1621.

Bookland EA, Swaminathan S, Oyasu R, Gilchrist KW, Lindstrom M, Reznikoff CA (1992b) Tumorigenic transformation and neoplastic progression of human uroepithelial cells after exposure in vitro to 4-aminobiphenyl or its metabolites. *Cancer Research*, **52**:1606–1614.

Bryant MS, Vineis P, Skipper PL, Tannenbaum SR (1988) Hemoglobin adducts of aromatic amines: Associations with smoking status and type of tobacco. *Proceedings of the National Academy of Sciences of the United States of America*, **85**:9788–9791.

Burger MS, Torino JL, Swaminathan S (2001) DNA damage in human transitional cell carcinoma cells after exposure to the proximate metabolite of the bladder carcinogen 4-aminobiphenyl. *Environmental and Molecular Mutagenesis*, **38**:1–11.

Butler MA, Guengerich FP, Kadlubar FF (1989a) Metabolic oxidation of the carcinogens 4-aminobiphenyl and 4,4′-methylene-bis(2-chloroaniline) by human hepatic microsomes and by purified rat hepatic cytochrome P-450 monooxygenases. *Cancer Research*, **49**:25–31.

Butler MA, Iwasaki M, Guengerich FP, Kadlubar FF (1989b) Human cytochrome P-450PA (P-450IA2), the phenacetin *O*-deethylase, is primarily responsible for the hepatic 3-demethylation of caffeine and *N*-oxidation of carcinogenic arylamines. *Proceedings of the National Academy of Sciences of the United States of America*, **86**:7696–7700.

Cairns P, Proctor AJ, Knowles MA (1991) Loss of heterozygosity at the *RB* locus is frequent and correlates with muscle invasion in bladder carcinoma. *Oncogene*, **6**:2305–2309.

Cairns T (1979) The ED_{01} study: Introduction, objectives, and experimental design. *Journal of Environmental Pathology and Toxicology*, **3**:1–7.

Cartwright RA, Rogers HJ, Barham-Hall D, Glashan RW, Ahmad RA, Higgins E, Kahn MA (1982) Role of *N*-acetyltransferase phenotypes in bladder carcinogenesis: A pharmacogenetic epidemiological approach to bladder cancer. *Lancet*, **16**:842–846.

Cascorbi I, Roots I, Brockmoller J (2001) Association of *NAT1* and *NAT2* polymorphisms to urinary bladder cancer: Significantly reduced risk in subjects with *NAT1*10*. *Cancer Research*, **61**:5051–5056.

Castelao JE, Yuan JM, Skipper PL, Tannenbaum SR, Gago-Dominguez M, Crowder JS, Ross RK, Yu MC (2001) Gender- and smoking-related bladder cancer risk. *Journal of the National Cancer Institute*, **93**:538–545.

Chou HC, Lang NP, Kadlubar FF (1995) Metabolic activation of the *N*-hydroxy derivative of the carcinogen 4-aminobiphenyl by human tissue sulfotransferases. *Carcinogenesis*, **16**:413–417.

Clayson DB, Lawson TA, Santana S, Bonser GM (1965) Correlation between the chemical induction of hyperplasia and of malignancy in the bladder epithelium. *British Journal of Cancer*, **19**:297–310.

Clayson DB, Lawson TA, Pringle JAS (1967) The carcinogenic action of 2-aminodiphenylene oxide and 4-aminodiphenyl on the bladder and liver of C57 × IF mouse. *British Journal of Cancer*, **1**:755–762.

Coghlin J, Gann PH, Hammond SK, Skipper PL, Taghizadeh K, Paul M, Tannenbaum SR (1991) 4-Aminobiphenyl hemoglobin adducts in fetuses exposed to the tobacco smoke carcinogen in utero. *Journal of the National Cancer Institute*, **83**:274–280.

Cohen SM (1995) The role of urinary physiology and chemistry in bladder carcinogenesis. *Food and Chemical Toxicology*, **33**:715–730.

Cohen SM, Ellwein LB (1990) Proliferative and genotoxic cellular effects in 2-acetylaminofluorene bladder and liver carcinogenesis: Biological modeling of the ED_{01} study. *Toxicology and Applied Pharmacology*, **104**:79–93.

Cordon-Cardo C, Reuter VE (1997) Alterations of tumor suppressor genes in bladder cancer. *Seminars in Diagnostic Pathology*, **14**:123–132.

Curigliano G, Zhang YJ, Wang LY, Flamini G, Alcini A, Ratto C, Giustacchini M, Alcini E, Cittadini A, Santella RM (1996) Immunohistochemical quantitation of 4-aminobiphenyl–DNA adducts and p53 nuclear overexpression in T1 bladder cancer of smokers and nonsmokers. *Carcinogenesis*, **17**:911–916.

Dang LN, McQueen CA (1999) Mutagenicity of 4-aminobiphenyl and 4-acetylbiphenyl in *Salmonella typhimurium* strains expressing different levels of N-acetyltransferase. *Toxicology and Applied Pharmacology*, **159**:77–82.

Deichmann WB, MacDonald WE (1968) The non-carcinogenicity of a single dose of 4-aminobiphenyl in the dog. *Food and Cosmetics Toxicology*, **6**:143–146.

Deichmann WB, Radomski JL, Anderson WAD, Coplan MM, Woods FM (1958) The carcinogenic action of *p*-aminobiphenyl in the dog; final report. *Industrial Medicine and Surgery*, **27**:25–26.

Deichmann WB, Radomski JL, Glass E, Anderson WAD, Coplan M, Woods FM (1965) Synergism among oral carcinogens. Simultaneous feeding of four bladder carcinogens to dogs. *Industrial Medicine and Surgery*, **34**:640–649.

Delclos KB, Miller DW, Lay JO Jr, Casciano DA, Walker RP, Fu PP, Kadlubar FF (1987) Identification of C8-modified deoxyinosine and N2- and C8-modified deoxyguanosine as major products of the in vitro reaction of *N*-hydroxy-6-aminochrysene with DNA and the formation of these adducts in isolated rat hepatocytes treated with 6-nitrochrysene and 6-aminochrysene. *Carcinogenesis*, **8**:1703–1709.

Del Santo P, Moneti G, Salvadori M, Saltutti C, Delle RA, Dolara P (1991) Levels of the adducts of 4-aminobiphenyl to hemoglobin in control subjects and bladder carcinoma patients. *Cancer Letters*, **60**:245–251.

Doerge DR, Churchwell MI, Marques MM, Beland FA (1999) Quantitative analyses of 4-aminobiphenyl–C8-deoxyguanosyl DNA adducts produced in vitro and in vivo using HPLC-ES-MS. *Carcinogenesis*, **6**:1055–1061.

Dooley KL, Stavenuiter JF, Westra JG, Kadlubar FF (1988) Comparative carcinogenicity of the food pyrolysis product, 2-amino-5-phenylpyridine, and the known human carcinogen, 4-aminobiphenyl, in the neonatal B6C3F1 mouse. *Cancer Letters*, **41**:99–103.

Dooley KL, Von Tungeln LS, Bucci T, Fu PP, Kadlubar FF (1992) Comparative carcinogenicity of 4-aminobiphenyl and the food pyrolysates, Glu-P-1, IQ, PhIP, and MeIQx in the neonatal B6C3F1 male mouse. *Cancer Letters*, **62**:205–209.

Eaton DL, Gallagher EP, Bammler TK, Kunze KL (1995) Role of cytochrome P4501A2 in chemical carcinogenesis: Implications for human variability in expression and enzyme activity. *Pharmacogenetics*, **5**:259–274.

Faraglia B, Chen SY, Gammon MD, Zhang Y, Teitelbaum SL, Neugut AI, Ahsan H, Garbowski GC, Hibshoosh H, Lin D, Kadlubar FF, Santella RM (2003) Evaluation of 4-aminobiphenyl–DNA adducts in human breast cancer: The influence of tobacco smoke. *Carcinogenesis*, **24**:719–725.

Feng Z, Hu W, Rom WN, Beland FA, Tang MS (2002) *N*-Hydroxy-4-aminobiphenyl–DNA binding in human *p53* gene: Sequence preference and the effect of C5 cytosine methylation. *Biochemistry*, **41**:6414–6421.

Flamini G, Romano G, Curigliano G, Chiominto A, Capelli G, Boninsegna A, Signorelli C, Ventura L, Santella RM, Sgambato A, Cittadini A (1998) 4-Aminobiphenyl–DNA adducts in laryngeal tissue and smoking habits: An immunohistochemical study. *Carcinogenesis*, **19**:353–357.

Flammang TJ, Kadlubar FF (1986) Acetyl coenzyme A-dependent metabolic activation of *N*-hydroxy-3,2′-dimethyl-4-aminobiphenyl and several carcinogenic *N*-hydroxy arylamines in relation to tissue and species differences, other acyl donors, and arylhydroxamic acid-dependent acyltransferases. *Carcinogenesis*, **7**:919–926.

Flammang TJ, Couch LH, Levy GN, Weber WW, Wise CK (1992) DNA adduct levels in congenic rapid and slow acetylator mouse strains following chronic administration of 4-aminobiphenyl. *Carcinogenesis*, **13**:1887–1891.

Fletcher K, Tinwell H, Ashby J (1998) Mutagenicity of the human bladder carcinogen 4-aminobiphenyl to the bladder of Muta™Mouse transgenic mice. *Mutation Research*, **400**:245–250.

Frederickson SM, Hatcher JF, Reznikoff CA, Swaminathan S (1992) Acetyl transferase-mediated metabolic activation of *N*-hydroxy-4-aminobiphenyl by human uroepithelial cells. *Carcinogenesis*, **13**:955–961.

Fretland AJ, Doll MA, Gray K, Feng Y, Hein DW (1997) Cloning, sequencing, and recombinant expression of NAT1, NAT2, and NAT3 derived from the C3H/HeJ (rapid) and A/HeJ (slow) acetylator inbred mouse: Functional characterization of the activation and deactivation of aromatic amine carcinogens. *Toxicology and Applied Pharmacology*, **142**:360–366.

Gaylor DW (1979) The ED$_{01}$ study: Summary and conclusions. *Journal of Environmental Pathology and Toxicology*, **3**:179–183.

Gorrod JW, Carter RL, Roe FJ (1968) Induction of hepatomas by 4-aminobiphenyl and three of its hydroxylated derivatives administered to newborn mice. *Journal of the National Cancer Institute*, **41**:403–410.

Hammons GJ, Guengerich FP, Weis CC, Beland FA, Kadlubar FF (1985) Metabolic oxidation of carcinogenic arylamines by rat, dog, and human hepatic microsomes and by purified flavin-containing and cytochrome P-450 monooxygenases. *Cancer Research*, **45**:3578–3585.

Hatcher JF, Swaminathan S (1992) Microsome-mediated transacetylation and binding of *N*-hydroxy-4-aminobiphenyl to nucleic acids by hepatic and bladder tissues from dog. *Carcinogenesis*, **13**:1705–1711.

Hatcher JF, Swaminathan S (1995) Detection of deoxyadenosine-4-aminobiphenyl adduct in DNA of human uroepithelial cells treated with *N*-hydroxy-4-aminobiphenyl following nuclease P1 enrichment and ^{32}P-postlabeling analysis. *Carcinogenesis*, **16**:295–301.

Hatcher JF, Swaminathan S (2002) Identification of *N*-(deoxyguanosin-8-yl)-4-azobiphenyl by ^{32}P-postlabeling analyses of DNA in human uroepithelial cells exposed to proximate metabolites of the environmental carcinogen 4-aminobiphenyl. *Environmental and Molecular Mutagenesis*, **39**:314–322.

Hatcher JF, Rao KP, Swaminathan S (1993) Mutagenic activation of 4-aminobiphenyl and its *N*-hydroxy derivatives by microsomes from cultured human uroepithelial cells. *Mutagenesis*, **8**:113–120.

Hein DW (1988) Acetylator genotype and arylamine-induced carcinogenesis. *Biochimica et Biophysica Acta*, **948**:37–66.

Hein DW, Grant DM, Sim E (2000) *Arylamine* N-*acetyltransferase (NAT) nomenclature* (http://louisville.edu/medschool/pharmacology/NAT.html).

Hickman ES, Moroni MC, Helin K (2002) The role of p53 and pRB in apoptosis and cancer. *Current Opinion in Genetics and Development*, **12**:60–66.

Hill AB (1965) The environment and disease: Association or causation? *Proceedings of the Royal Society of Medicine*, **58**:295–300.

Hughes MF, Smith BJ, Eling TE (1992) The oxidation of 4-aminobiphenyl by horseradish peroxidase. *Chemical Research in Toxicology*, **5**:340–345.

IARC (1972) 4-Aminobiphenyl. In: *Some inorganic substances, chlorinated hydrocarbons, aromatic amines,* N-*nitroso compounds, and natural products*. Lyon, International Agency for Research on Cancer, pp. 74–79 (IARC Monographs on the Evaluation of Carcinogenic Risks to Humans, Vol. 1).

IARC (1986) *Tobacco smoking*. Lyon, International Agency for Research on Cancer, 421 pp. (IARC Monographs on the Evaluation of Carcinogenic Risks to Humans, Vol. 38).

IARC (1987) 4-Aminobiphenyl (Group 1). In: *Overall evaluations of carcinogenicity: An updating of IARC Monographs Volumes 1 to 42*. Lyon, International Agency for Research on Cancer, pp. 91–92 (IARC Monographs on the Evaluation of Carcinogenic Risks to Humans, Supplement 7).

Ioachim E, Charchanti A, Stavropoulos NE, Skopelitou A, Athanassiou ED, Agnantis NJ (2000) Immunohistochemical expression of retinoblastoma gene product (Rb), p53 protein, MDM2, c-erbB-2, HLA-DR and proliferation indices in human urinary bladder carcinoma. *Histology and Histopathology*, **15**:721–727.

Ishikawa J, Xu HJ, Hu SX, Yandell DW, Maeda S, Kamidono S, Benedict WF, Takahashi R (1991) Inactivation of the retinoblastoma gene in human bladder and renal cell carcinomas. *Cancer Research*, **51**:5736–5743.

Kadlubar FF, Miller JA, Miller EC (1977) Hepatic microsomal *N*-glucuronidation and nucleic acid binding of *N*-hydroxy arylamines in relation to urinary bladder carcinogenesis. *Cancer Research*, **37**:805–814.

Kadlubar FF, Frederick CB, Weis CD, Zenser TV (1982) Prostaglandin endoperoxide synthetase-mediated metabolism of carcinogenic aromatic amines and their binding to DNA and protein. *Biochemical and Biophysical Research Communications*, **108**:253–258.

Kadlubar FF, Dooley KL, Teitel CH, Roberts DW, Benson RW, Butler MA, Bailey JR, Young JF, Skipper PW, Tannenbaum SR (1991) Frequency of urination and its effects on metabolism, pharmacokinetics, blood hemoglobin adduct formation, and liver and urinary bladder DNA adduct levels in beagle dogs given the carcinogen 4-aminobiphenyl. *Cancer Research*, **51**:4371–4377.

Kimura S, Kawabe M, Ward JM, Morishima H, Kadlubar FF, Hammons GJ, Fernandez-Salguero P, Gonzalez FJ (1999) CYP1A2 is not the primary enzyme responsible for 4-aminobiphenyl-induced hepatocarcinogenesis in mice. *Carcinogenesis*, **20**:1825–1830.

Koss LG, Melamed MR, Ricci A, Melick WF, Kelly RE (1965) Carcinogenesis in the human urinary bladder. Observations after exposure to *para*-aminodiphenyl. *New England Journal of Medicine*, **272**:767–770.

Koss LG, Melamed MR, Kelly RE (1969) Further cytologic and histologic studies of bladder lesions in workers exposed to *para*-aminodiphenyl: Progress report. *Journal of the National Cancer Institute*, **43**:233–243.

Kriek E (1992) Fifty years of research on *N*-acetyl-2-aminofluorene, one of the most versatile compounds in experimental research. *Journal of Cancer Research and Clinical Oncology*, **118**:481–489.

Lakshmi VM, Mattammal MB, Zenser TV, Davis BB (1990) Mechanism of peroxidative activation of the bladder carcinogen 2-amino-4-(5-nitro-2-furyl)-thiazole (ANFT): Comparison with benzidine. *Carcinogenesis*, **11**:1965–1970.

Lang M, Pelkonen O (1999) Metabolism of xenobiotics and chemical carcinogenesis. *IARC Scientific Publications*, **148**:13–22.

Littlefield NA, Farmer JH, Gaylor DW, Sheldon WG (1979) Effects of dose and time in a long-term, low-dose carcinogenic study. *Journal of Environmental Pathology and Toxicology*, **3**:17–34.

Logothetis CJ, Xu HJ, Ro JY, Hu SX, Sahin A, Ordonez N, Benedict WF (1992) Altered expression of retinoblastoma protein and known prognostic variables in locally advanced bladder cancer. *Journal of the National Cancer Institute*, **84**:1256–1261.

Lower GM Jr, Nilsson T, Nelson CE, Wolf H, Gamsky TE, Bryan GT (1979) *N*-Acetyltransferase phenotype and risk in urinary bladder cancer: Approaches in molecular epidemiology. Preliminary results in Sweden and Denmark. *Environmental Health Perspectives*, **29**:71–79.

Lu ML, Wikman F, Orntoft TF, Charytonowicz E, Rabbani F, Zhang Z, Dalbagni G, Pohar KS, Yu G, Cordon-Cardo C (2002) Impact of alterations affecting the p53 pathway in bladder cancer on clinical outcome, assessed by conventional and array-based methods. *Clinical Cancer Research*, **8**:171–179.

Manjanatha MG, Li EE, Fu PP, Heflich RH (1996) H- and K-*ras* mutational profiles in chemically induced liver tumours from B6C3F1 and CD-1 mice. *Journal of Toxicology and Environmental Health*, **47**:195–208.

Martone T, Airoldi L, Magagnotti C, Coda R, Randone D, Malaveille C, Avanzi G, Merletti F, Hautefeuille A, Vineis P (1998) 4-Aminobiphenyl–DNA adducts and *p53* mutations in bladder cancer. *International Journal of Cancer*, **75**:512–516.

Mattano SS, Land S, King CM, Weber WW (1989) Purification and biochemical characterization of hepatic arylamine *N*-acetyltransferase from rapid and slow acetylator mice: Identity with arylhydroxamic acid *N,O*-acyltransferase and *N*-hydroxyarylamine *O*-acetyltransferase. *Molecular Pharmacology*, **68**:599–609.

McQueen CA, Chau B, Erickson RP, Tjalkens RB, Philbert MA (2003) The effects of genetic variation in *N*-acetyltransferases on 4-aminobiphenyl genotoxicity in mouse liver. *Chemico-Biological Interactions*, **146**:51–60.

Melamed MR, Koss LG, Ricci A, Whitmore WF Jr (1960) Cytohistological observations on developing carcinoma of urinary bladder in man. *Cancer (Philadelphia)*, **13**:67–74.

Melick WF, Escue HM, Naryka JJ, Mezera RA, Wheeler EP (1955) The first reported cases of human bladder tumors due to a new carcinogen—Xenylamine. *Journal of Urology (Baltimore)*, **74**:760–766.

Melick WF, Naryka JJ, Kelly RE (1971) Bladder cancer due to exposure to *para*-aminobiphenyl: A 17-year follow-up. *Journal of Urology (Baltimore)*, **106**:220–226.

Merck (1998) *Merck veterinary manual*. Whitehouse Station, NJ, Merck & Co., Inc.

Miller JA, Miller EC (1977) Ultimate chemical carcinogens as reactive mutagenic electrophiles. In: Hiatt HH, Watson JD, Winsten JA, eds. *Origins of human cancer*. Cold Spring Harbor, NY, Cold Spring Harbor Laboratory, pp. 605–627.

Miller JA, Wyatt CS, Miller EC, Hartmann HA (1961) The *N*-hydroxylation of 4-acetylaminobiphenyl by the rat and dog and the strong carcinogenicity of *N*-hydroxy-4-acetylaminobiphenyl in the rat. *Cancer Research*, **21**:1465–1473.

Oda Y (2004) Analysis of the involvement of human *N*-acetyltransferase 1 in the genotoxic activation of bladder carcinogenic arylamines using a SOS/umu assay system. *Mutation Research*, **554**:399–406.

Oscarson M, Ingelman-Sundberg M, Daly AK, Nebert DW (n.d.) *Human Cytochrome P450 (CYP) Allele Nomenclature Committee* (http://www.cypalleles.ki.se/).

Parsons BL, Culp SJ, Manjanatha MG, Heflich RH (2002) Occurrence of H-*ras* codon 61 CAA to AAA mutation during mouse liver tumor progression. *Carcinogenesis*, **23**:943–948.

Parsons BL, Beland FA, Von Tungeln LS, Delongchamp RR, Fu P, Heflich RH (2005) Levels of 4-aminobiphenyl-induced somatic H-*ras* mutation in mouse liver correlate with potential for liver tumor development. *Molecular Carcinogenesis*, **42**:193–201.

Pauli BU, Alroy J, Weinstein RS (1983) The ultrastructure and pathobiology of urinary bladder cancer. In: Bryan GT, Cohen SM, eds. *The pathology of bladder cancer, Vol. II*. Boca Raton, FL, CRC Press, pp. 41–140.

Poirier MC, Beland FA (1992) DNA adduct measurements and tumor incidence during chronic carcinogen exposure in animal models: Implications for DNA adduct-based human cancer risk assessment. *Chemical Research in Toxicology*, **5**:749–755.

Poirier MC, Fullerton NF, Smith BA, Beland FA (1995) DNA adduct formation and tumorigenesis in mice during the chronic administration of 4-aminobiphenyl at multiple dose levels. *Carcinogenesis*, **16**:2917–2921.

Presti JCJ, Reuter VE, Galan T, Fair WR, Cordon-Cardo C (1991) Molecular genetic alterations in superficial and locally advanced human bladder cancer. *Cancer Research*, **51**:5405–5409.

Primdahl H, von der Maase H, Christensen M, Wolf H, Orntoft TF (2000) Allelic deletions of cell growth regulators during progression of bladder cancer. *Cancer Research*, **60**:6623–6629.

Reznikoff CA, Loretz LJ, Johnson MD, Swaminathan S (1986) Quantitative assessments of the cytotoxicity of bladder carcinogens towards cultured normal human uroepithelial cells. *Carcinogenesis*, **7**:1625–1632.

Roberts DW, Benson RW, Groopman JD, Flammang TJ, Nagle WA, Moss AJ, Kadlubar FF (1988) Immunochemical quantitation of DNA adducts derived from the human bladder carcinogen 4-aminobiphenyl. *Cancer Research*, **48**:6336–6342.

Sachse C, Bhambra U, Smith G, Lightfoot TJ, Barrett JH, Scollay J, Garner RC, Boobis AR, Wolf CR, Gooderham NJ, Colorectal Cancer Study Group (2003) Polymorphisms in the cytochrome P450 CYP1A2 gene (*CYP1A2*) in colorectal cancer patients and controls: Allele frequencies, linkage disequilibrium and influence on caffeine metabolism. *British Journal of Clinical Pharmacology*, **55**:68–76.

Sarkar MA, Nseyo UO, Zhong B-Z (2002) Mutagenic outcome of the urinary carcinogen 4-aminobiphenyl is increased in acidic pH. *Environmental Toxicology and Pharmacology*, **11**:23–26.

Schieferstein GJ, Littlefield NA, Gaylor DW, Sheldon WG, Burgers GT (1985) Carcinogenesis of 4-aminobiphenyl in BALB/cStCrlfC3Hf/Nctr mice. *European Journal of Cancer and Clinical Oncology*, **21**:865–873.

Schroeder JC, Conway K, Li Y, Mistry K, Bell DA, Taylor JA (2003) *p53* mutations in bladder cancer: Evidence for exogenous versus endogenous risk factors. *Cancer Research*, **63**:7530–7538.

Sesardic D, Boobis AR, Edwards RJ, Davies DS (1988) A form of cytochrome P450 in man, orthologous to form *d* in the rat, catalyses the *O*-deethylation of phenacetin and is inducible by cigarette smoking. *British Journal of Clinical Pharmacology*, **26**:363–372.

Skipper PL, Tannenbaum SR, Ross RK, Yu MC (2003) Nonsmoking-related arylamine exposure and bladder cancer risk. *Cancer Epidemiology, Biomarkers and Prevention*, **12**:503–507.

Smith BJ, Curtis JF, Eling TE (1991) Bioactivation of xenobiotics by prostaglandin H synthase. *Chemico-Biological Interactions*, **79**:245–264.

Sonich-Mullin C, Fielder R, Wiltse J, Baetcke K, Dempsey J, Fenner-Crisp P, Grant D, Hartley M, Knaap A, Krose D, Mangelsdorf I, Meek E, Rice JM, Younes M (2001) IPCS conceptual framework for evaluating a mode of action for chemical carcinogenesis. *Regulatory Toxicology and Pharmacology*, **34**:146–152.

Swaminathan S, Reznikoff CA (1992) Metabolism and nucleic acid binding of *N*-hydroxy-4-acetylaminobiphenyl and *N*-acetoxy-4-acetylaminobiphenyl by cultured human uroepithelial cells. *Cancer Research*, **52**:3286–3294.

Talaska G, Dooley KL, Kadlubar FF (1990) Detection and characterization of carcinogen–DNA adducts in exfoliated urothelial cells from 4-aminobiphenyl-treated dogs by ^{32}P-postlabelling and subsequent thin-layer and high-pressure liquid chromatography. *Carcinogenesis*, **11**:639–646.

Tiguert R, Bianco FJJ, Oskanian P, Li Y, Grignon DJ, Wood DPJ, Pontes JE, Sarkar FH (2001) Structural alteration of p53 protein in patients with muscle invasive bladder transitional cell carcinoma. *Journal of Urology*, **166**:2155–2160.

Tsuneoka Y, Dalton TP, Miller ML, Clay CD, Shertzer HG, Talaska G, Medvedovic M, Nebert DW (2003) 4-Aminobiphenyl-induced liver and urinary bladder DNA adduct formation in Cyp1a2(−/−) and Cyp1a2(+/+) mice. *Journal of the National Cancer Institute*, **95**:1227–1237.

Underwood PM, Zhou Q, Jaeger M, Reilman R, Pinney S, Warshawsky D, Talaska G (1997) Chronic, topical administration of 4-aminobiphenyl induces tissue-specific DNA adducts in mice. *Toxicology and Applied Pharmacology*, **144**:325–331.

Verghis SBM, Essigmann JM, Kadlubar FF, Morningstar ML, Lasko DD (1997) Specificity of mutagenesis by 4-aminobiphenyl: Mutations at G residues in bacteriophage M13 DNA and G → C transversions at a unique dG$^{8\text{-ABP}}$ lesion in single-stranded DNA. *Carcinogenesis*, **18**:2403–2414.

Vineis P, Caporaso N, Tannenbaum SR, Skipper PL, Glogowski J, Bartsch H, Coda M, Talaska G, Kadlubar FF (1990) Acetylation phenotype, carcinogen–hemoglobin adducts, and cigarette smoking. *Cancer Research*, **50**:3002–3004.

Von Tungeln LS, Bucci TJ, Hart RW, Kadlubar FF, Fu PP (1996) Inhibitory effect of caloric restriction on tumorigenicity induced by 4-aminobiphenyl and 2-amino-1-methyl-6-phenylimidazo-[4,5-b]pyridine (PhIP) in the CD1 newborn mouse bioassay. *Cancer Letters*, **104**:133–136.

Vousden KH, Lu X (2002) Live or let die: The cell's response to p53. *Nature Reviews. Cancer*, **2**:594–604.

Walpole AL, Williams MHC, Roberts DC (1952) The carcinogenic action of 4-aminodiphenyl and 3:2′-dimethyl-4-aminodiphenyl. *British Journal of Industrial Medicine*, **9**:255–263.

Walpole AL, Williams MHC, Roberts DC (1954) Tumours of the urinary bladder in dogs after ingestion of 4-aminodiphenyl. *British Journal of Industrial Medicine*, **11**:105–109.

Weston A, Caporaso NE, Taghizadeh K, Hoover RN, Tannenbaum SR, Skipper PL, Resau JH, Trump BF, Harris CC (1991) Measurement of 4-aminobiphenyl–hemoglobin adducts in lung cancer cases and controls. *Cancer Research*, **51**:5219–5223.

Wright C, Thomas D, Mellon K, Neal DE, Horne CH (1995) Expression of retinoblastoma gene product and p53 protein in bladder carcinoma: Correlation with Ki67 index. *British Journal of Urology*, **75**:173–179.

Wu XR, Lin JH, Walz T, Haner M, Yu J, Aebi U, Sun TT (1994) Mammalian uroplakins. A group of highly conserved urothelial differentiation-related membrane proteins. *Journal of Biological Chemistsy*, **269**:13716–13724.

FORMALDEHYDE AND GLUTARALDEHYDE AND NASAL CYTOTOXICITY: CASE-STUDY WITHIN THE CONTEXT OF THE IPCS FRAMEWORK FOR ANALYSING THE RELEVANCE OF A CANCER MODE OF ACTION FOR HUMANS[1]

Douglas McGregor, Hermann Bolt, Vincent Cogliano, & Hans-Bernhard Richter-Reichhelm

Formaldehyde and glutaraldehyde cause toxicity to the nasal epithelium of rats and mice upon inhalation. In addition, formaldehyde above certain concentrations induces dose-related increases in nasal tumours in rats and mice, but glutaraldehyde does not. Using the 2006 International Programme on Chemical Safety (IPCS) human framework for the analysis of cancer mode of action (MOA), an MOA for formaldehyde was formulated and its relevance tested against the properties of the non-carcinogenic glutaraldehyde. These compounds produce similar patterns of response in histopathology and in genotoxicity tests (although formaldehyde has been much more extensively studied). The MOA is based on the induction of sustained cytotoxicity and reparative cell proliferation induced by formaldehyde at concentrations that also induce nasal tumours upon long-term exposure. Data on dose dependency and temporal relationships of key events are consistent with this MOA. While a genotoxic MOA can never be ruled out for a compound that is clearly genotoxic, at least in vitro, the non-genotoxic properties fundamental to the proposed MOA can explain the neoplastic response in the nose and may be more informative than genotoxicity in risk assessment. It is not yet fully explained why glutaraldehyde remains non-carcinogenic upon inhalation, but its greater inherent toxicity may be a key factor. The dual aldehyde functions in glutaraldehyde are likely to produce damage resulting in fewer kinetic possibilities (particularly for proteins involved in differentiation control) and lower potential for repair (nucleic acids) than would be the case for formaldehyde. While there have been few studies of possible glutaraldehyde-associated cancer, the evidence that formaldehyde is a human carcinogen is strong for nasopharyngeal cancers, although less so for sinonasal cancers. This apparent discrepancy could be due in part to the classification of human nasal tumours with tumours of the sinuses, which would receive much less exposure to inhaled formaldehyde. Evaluation of the human relevance of the proposed MOA of formaldehyde in rodents is restricted by human data limitations, although the key events are plausible. It is clear that the human relevance of the formaldehyde MOA in rodents cannot be excluded on either kinetic or dynamic grounds.

INTRODUCTION

Formaldehyde and glutaraldehyde are aliphatic mono- and dialdehydes, respectively, that undergo reactions typical of aldehydes to form acetals, cyanohydrins, oximes, hydrazones, and bisulfite complexes. They are highly reactive chemicals and produce covalently cross-linked complexes with DNA and proteins. Their metabolism has some commonality in that they are both oxidized by aldehyde dehydrogenases. Several studies have demonstrated that inhalation exposure to formaldehyde causes nasal tumours in rats, whereas no nasal tumours were observed in the only 2-year inhalation study of rats exposed to glutaraldehyde.

---

[1] This article, to which WHO owns copyright, was originally published in 2006 in *Critical Reviews in Toxicology*, Volume 36, pages 821–835. It has been edited for this WHO publication and includes corrigenda.

Formaldehyde

Formaldehyde has been tested for carcinogenicity by the inhalation route in mice, rats, and Syrian hamsters, by oral administration (drinking-water) in rats, by skin application in mice, and by subcutaneous injection in rats. There is conclusive evidence from the inhalation studies that formaldehyde is a carcinogen in rats.

There is considerable evidence that prolonged inhalation exposure to formaldehyde induces highly non-linear dose-related increases in the incidence of tumours of the anterior and posterior lateral meatus of rats (Morgan et al., 1986; Feron et al., 1988; Woutersen et al., 1989; Monticello et al., 1996; Kamata et al., 1997; CIIT, 1999). There are sharp increases in tumour incidence at formaldehyde concentrations equal to and greater than 7.2 mg/m^3. Exposure to concentrations of 2.4 mg/m^3 and lower induced no malignant nasal tumours. Table 1 combines the data from two published rat studies (Kerns et al., 1983a; Monticello et al., 1996) conducted at the same laboratory and some additional information from one of these studies on a number of rats that had not been examined at the time of the publications (Schlosser et al., 2003). The majority of formaldehyde-induced neoplasms were squamous cell carcinomas.

Table 1. Combined incidence of nasal squamous cell carcinomas in rats exposed to formaldehyde.

Formaldehyde concentration (mg/m^3)	Number of rats at risk[a]	Actual number of tumours[b]
0	122	0
0.84	27	0
2.4	126	0
7.2	113	3
12	34	22
18	182	157

Note: Adapted from Schlosser et al. (2003).
[a] Rats at risk are those that survived to 2 years and were examined at that time plus those that died before 2 years in which tumours were found.
[b] Rats in which tumours were found at or before 2 years.

In contrast, inhalation studies in Syrian hamsters showed no carcinogenic effect at a single dose of 12.3 mg/m^3 (Dalbey, 1982), and one of two inhalation studies in mice showed no effect in females and squamous cell carcinomas in 2/17 males killed at 2 years at a high-dose concentration of 17.6 mg/m^3 (Kerns et al., 1983a, 1983b), whereas the other was inadequate for evaluation (Horton et al., 1963).

Studies on rats using other routes of exposure produced no significant results in two of four drinking-water studies (Takahashi et al., 1986; Tobe et al., 1989), forestomach papillomas in one study (Til et al., 1989), and leukaemia and gastrointestinal tract tumours in another (Soffritti et al., 1989), but the interpretation of the last study has been questioned (Feron et al., 1990). Mouse skin application and subcutaneous injection studies were not suitable for evaluation. In no study in rodents was there a significant increase in nasal tumours other than in the five inhalation exposure studies in rats—that is, at the entry portal.

Glutaraldehyde

Glutaraldehyde has been tested for carcinogenicity by the inhalation route in mice and rats and by oral administration (drinking-water) in rats. Inhalation studies showed no carcinogenic effect in either B6C3F1 mice exposed to a single concentration of 400 $\mu g/m^3$ for 78 weeks (Zissu et al., 1998) or multiple concentrations up to 1000 $\mu g/m^3$ for 2 years (NTP, 1999) or F344 rats exposed to concentrations of up to 3000 $\mu g/m^3$ for 2 years (NTP, 1999). In a drinking-water study in which male and female F344 rats were exposed to glutaraldehyde concentrations of up to 4000 mg/m^3 for 2 years, increased incidences of large granular cell lymphatic leukaemia were found in the spleen of females at all exposure concentrations (Ballantyne, 1995; Van Miller et al., 1995).

1. IS THE WEIGHT OF EVIDENCE SUFFICIENT TO ESTABLISH A MODE OF ACTION (MOA) IN ANIMALS?

A. Postulated mode of action

Prolonged exposure to formaldehyde above a critical concentration induces sustained cytotoxicity and cell proliferation. As a result of genetic changes within this proliferating cell population, neoplasia emerges. The genetic changes are postulated to be secondary to the cytotoxicity, metaplasia, and hyperplasia that are clearly induced by formaldehyde. Formaldehyde is a genotoxic substance in vitro and forms DNA–protein cross-links (DPX). DPX are a well established indicator of formaldehyde exposure, but it is not clear whether they are premutational lesions required to produce neoplasia (by initiating DNA replication errors, resulting in mutation). Apart from the abundance of DPX observations in rats, there is little evidence that formaldehyde is mutagenic to mammalian cells in vivo.

This postulated MOA is mainly based on observations of consistent, non-linear dose–response relationships for all three key events (sustained cell proliferation, DPX, and tumours) and concordance of incidence of these effects across regions of the nasal passages.

B. Key events

Formaldehyde

Limitation of damage to the entry portal following exposure to formaldehyde is clearly important, with metabolism playing a significant role in the process. The importance of the entry portal for formaldehyde-induced nasal tumours is supported by the observation that the principal non-neoplastic effect in rats exposed orally to formaldehyde solutions is the development of histological changes within the forestomach and glandular stomach (Til et al., 1989; Tobe et al., 1989).

Formaldehyde is an endogenous metabolic product of *N*-, *O*-, and *S*-demethylation reactions within cells (Hardman et al., 2001), and circulating concentrations of about 2.0–2.6 $\mu g/g$ blood are normal in unexposed mammals (Heck et al., 1982, 1985; Casanova et al., 1988). Exogenous formaldehyde is rapidly detoxified upon absorption. It has a half-life in plasma of about 1 min in rats exposed intravenously (Rietbrock, 1965), and it readily and spontaneously combines with reduced glutathione to form *S*-hydroxymethylglutathione, the substrate for alcohol dehydrogenase 3 (ADH3, also known as glutathione-dependent formaldehyde dehydrogenase) (Uotila & Koivusalo, 1974; Koivusalo et al., 1989), to form *S*-formylgluta-thione, which is further metabolized to formic acid and reduced glutathione by *S*-formyl-glutathione hydrolase (Uotila & Koivusalo, 1997). The K_M for initial binding of hydroxy-methylglutathione with ADH3 is about 0.004 mmol/l, and the concentration of free formal-dehyde is likely to be even lower (Uotila & Koivusalo, 1997; Hedberg et al., 1998). It may be toxicologically significant that formaldehyde also combines with thiols such as cysteine and cysteinylglycine (Holmquist & Vallee, 1991). In addition to this efficient metabolic detoxification mechanism, the mucociliary apparatus provides protection of the underlying epithelium from gases and vapours. Thus, in order to attain free formaldehyde concentrations that may be cytotoxic to the target tissue, relatively high concentrations of formaldehyde vapour must be delivered to the target site to overcome these protective mechanisms. Mech-anistic events of clear significance for carcinogenicity occur at dose levels where formal-dehyde detoxification mechanisms are saturated in rats (Casanova & Heck, 1987).

The predominant non-neoplastic and preneoplastic events that have been measured and associated with nasal cancer formation following inhalation exposure of the nasal epithelium to formaldehyde include cytotoxicity, DPX formation, nasal epithelial cell regenerative pro-liferation, squamous metaplasia, and inflammation, which are site-specific, highly non-linear response processes in concordance with the incidence of nasal tumours.

The relative magnitude of an increase in cell proliferation is dependent upon the size of the target cell population within specific regions of the nasal cavity and not always directly related to the length of exposure, or total cumulative exposure (Swenberg et al., 1983, 1986; Monticello et al., 1991, 1996; Monticello & Morgan, 1994). These factors have been well defined and measured in a number of studies in rat, monkey, and human epithelial cells. In a 24-month carcinogenicity assay with interim sacrifices at 3, 6, 12, and 18 months, cell proliferation was demonstrated in rats exposed to 7.2, 12, and 18 mg/m^3 at all times (Monticello et al., 1991, 1996).

An immunohistochemical technique was used to assess the presence of p53 protein, a marker of cell proliferation (proliferating cell nuclear antigen, or PCNA), and tumour growth factor (TGF)-α in the histopathological sections of the same tumours. In addition to the p53-positive immunostaining in squamous cell carcinomas, especially in cells with keratinization, p53-positive immunostaining was observed in preneoplastic hyperkeratotic plaques, while normal nasal mucosa did not stain. A correlation was found between the distribution of immunostaining of PCNA and that of p53 (Wolf et al., 1995).

The formation of DPX in rats is a non-linear function of concentration (Casanova & Heck, 1987; Casanova et al., 1989, 1994; Heck & Casanova, 1995) and correlates with the site specificity of tumours (Casanova et al., 1994). Cross-links were not detected in the olfactory mucosa or in the bone marrow of rats (Casanova-Schmitz et al., 1984; Casanova & Heck, 1987). DPX have been found in rhesus monkeys following inhalation exposure to formal-dehyde, with the highest concentrations in the middle turbinates, followed by the anterior lateral wall septum and nasopharynx (Casanova et al., 1991).

Studies of rats, mice, Syrian hamsters, and rhesus monkeys exposed to formaldehyde for 13 (mice) or 26 weeks found that squamous metaplasia in the nasal turbinates developed in rats and rhesus monkeys at 3.7 mg/m^3, but not in Syrian hamsters or, at 4.9 mg/m^3, in mice (Rusch et al., 1983; Maronpot et al., 1986). Cell replication is also a feature of the more tumour-susceptible areas of the nasal epithelium of rats (Casanova et al., 1994).

Glutaraldehyde

Inhalation exposure to glutaraldehyde at 400 µg/m^3 for 78 weeks resulted in non-neoplastic lesions in the nasal vestibule of female mice, consisting of hyperplasia of the squamous epithelium lining the dorsal wall and the lateral aspect of the atrioturbinate (Zissu et al., 1998).

In the United States National Toxicology Program (NTP) studies of glutaraldehyde, the nasal changes observed in male and female rats included the following:

1. In the squamous epithelium in the most rostral part of the nasal passage, behind the external nares, there were increased incidences of hyperplasia and inflammation. The hyperplasia was a minimal to marked change characterized by variable thickening of the epithelium due to an increase in the number of cell layers and, in the more severe cases, varying degrees of keratin accumulation.
2. In the respiratory epithelium, there was hyperplasia, minimal goblet cell hyperplasia (primarily along the nasal septum and ventral meatus), inflammation, and squamous metaplasia, with accumulation of keratin on the epithelial surface in the more severe cases.
3. In the olfactory epithelium of the dorsal meatus, there were slightly increased incidences of hyaline degeneration.

The glutaraldehyde-associated inflammation that was observed in the squamous epithelial and respiratory epithelial regions was a minimal to marked change consisting of multifocal to locally extensive infiltrates of neutrophils, lymphocytes, and plasma cells. Occasionally, there were a few macrophages within the lamina propria and, in severe cases, within the epithelium itself. In male and female mice of this same study, the lesions were qualitatively similar to those found in rats. Females were more severely affected than male mice.

Glutaraldehyde induced DPX in a TK6 human lymphoblast cell line (St. Clair et al., 1991). In vivo, glutaraldehyde induced cell proliferation (S-phase nuclei) in nasal cells in rats and mice exposed by inhalation (Gross et al., 1994) and nasal instillation (St. Clair et al., 1990). In a parallel nasal instillation study by the same authors, formaldehyde induced the same level of cell proliferation at 20-fold higher molar concentrations.

C. Dose–response relationship

Formaldehyde

Available data from rats exposed to formaldehyde show a highly non-linear dose–response pattern for the key events, with no observed effects at 2.4 mg/m^3, a minimal response at 7.2 mg/m^3, and a sharp increase at 12 and 18 mg/m^3.

In rats exposed to formaldehyde, no increases in cell turnover or DNA synthesis were found in the nasal mucosa after subchronic or chronic exposure to concentrations of ≤ 2.4 mg/m^3 (Rusch et al., 1983; Zwart et al., 1988; Monticello et al., 1991; Casanova et al., 1994). Small, site-specific increases in the rate of cell turnover were noted at 3.7 mg/m^3 (6 h/day, 5 days/week, for 13 weeks) in Wistar rats (Zwart et al., 1988) and in the rate of DNA synthesis at 7.2 mg/m^3 in Fischer 344 rats exposed for a similar period (Casanova et al., 1994). At these concentrations, however, an adaptive response would seem to occur in rat nasal epithelium, since cell turnover rates after 6 weeks (Monticello et al., 1991) or 13 weeks (Zwart et al., 1988) are lower than those after 1–4 days of exposure. The unit length labelling index (ULLI) method was used to establish the proliferation in male Fischer 344 rats exposed to formaldehyde concentrations of 0, 0.84, 2.4, 7.2, 12, or 18 mg/m^3 for 6 h/day, 5 days/week, for 3, 6, 12, 18, or 24 months. Significant increases in ULLI were present only in the 12 and 18 mg/m^3 groups, with the greater increases on the anterior lateral meatus and the medial maxilloturbinate. Elevated ULLI in the anterior dorsal septum developed later in the course of the exposure. This belated elevation of ULLI may have been secondary to changes in airflow patterns and thus local formaldehyde concentrations associated with growth of lesions and distortion of the airspace in those areas of the nose more susceptible to neoplasia (Monticello et al., 1996).

The non-linear relationships for formaldehyde-induced DPX formation, epithelial cell proliferation, and subsequently nasal tumours are demonstrated in Table 2. It is arguable that the designations of high- and low-tumour areas proposed by Casanova et al. (1994) are not the most appropriate, and consequently the truly high tumour incidence region DPX response may have been diluted by that of the intermediate tumour incidence (posterior lateral meatus) region.

Other studies showed that Fischer 344 rats exposed to 1.2 mg/m^3 (22 h/day, 7 days/week, for 26 weeks) developed no detectable nasal lesions, whereas at 3.6 mg/m^3, the only histological change was squamous metaplasia in the nasal turbinates (Rusch et al., 1983). The development of mild squamous metaplasia was similarly demonstrated in the nasal turbinates of Fischer 344 rats exposed to 2.4 mg/m^3 (6 h/day, 5 days/week, for 24 months) (Kerns et al., 1983b). Epithelial dysplasia and rhinitis were also observed in these rats. The occurrence of squamous metaplasia appears to be the histological feature requiring the lowest formaldehyde concentration of any of the in vivo responses reported.

A rat, anatomically accurate computational fluid dynamics model was used to test whether the distribution of formaldehyde-induced squamous metaplasia was related to the location of high-flux regions posterior to the squamous epithelium. Squamous metaplasia was considered present when $\geq 50\%$ of a subsection was lined by squamous epithelium. No squamous metaplasia was present in sections of nose from rats exposed to 2.4 mg/m^3 or less. Squamous metaplasia was present on the lateral meatus after exposure to 7.2 mg/m^3 or more and on the lateral and medial walls of the airway after exposure to 12 or 18 mg/m^3 (Kimbell et al., 1997).

There is evidence that glutathione-mediated detoxification of formaldehyde within nasal tissues becomes saturated in rats at inhalation exposures above 4.8 mg/m^3. This saturation of formaldehyde metabolism may contribute to the non-linearity of the dose–response relationships for DPX, cell proliferation, and tumour incidence at exposures above this level (Casanova & Heck, 1987).

Table 2. Comparative effects of formaldehyde exposure upon cell proliferation, DNA–protein cross-linking, and tumour incidence.

Formalde-hyde concen-tration (mg/m^3)	Cell proliferation ($[^3H]$thymidine-labelled cells/mm basement membrane)[a]			DNA–protein cross-link formation (pmol $[^{14}C]$-formaldehyde bound/mg DNA)[b]		Incidence of nasal carcinoma[c]			
	Anterior lateral meatus	*Posterior lateral meatus*	*Anterior mid-septum*	*"High-tumour region"*	*"Low-tumour region"*	*All sites*	*Anterior lateral meatus*	*Posterior lateral meatus*	*Anterior mid-septum*
0	10.11	7.69	6.58	0	0	0/90	0/90	0/90	0/90
0.84	10.53	7.82	8.04	5	5	0/90	0/90	0/90	0/90
2.4	9.83	11.24	12.74	8	8	0/96	0/96	0/96	0/96
7.2	15.68	9.96	4.15	30	10	1/90	1/90	0/90	0/90
12	76.79	15.29	30.01	–	–	20/90	12/90	2/90	0/90
18	93.22	59.52	75.71	150	60	69/147	17/147	9/147	8/147

[a] Cell proliferation measured in three locations of the nasal epithelium in male F344 rats exposed to the indicated concentrations of formaldehyde, 6 h/day, 5 days/week, for 3 months (Monticello et al., 1996).

[b] Extent of DNA–protein cross-link formation measured in two regions of the nasal cavity (respiratory mucosa) in male F344 rats exposed to the indicated concentrations of formaldehyde, 6 h/day, 5 days/week, for about 12 weeks; the complete lateral meatus was designated the "high-tumour region"; the "low-tumour region" comprised the medial aspects of naso- and maxilloturbinates, posterior lateral wall, posterior dorsal septum excluding olfactory region, and nasopharyngeal meatuses (Casanova et al., 1994). Data were derived from graphical representations in the reference cited.

[c] Incidence of nasal tumours within the entire nasal cavity or the anterior lateral meatus, posterior lateral meatus, or anterior mid-septum in male F344 rats exposed to the indicated concentrations of formaldehyde, 6 h/day, 5 days/week, for 24 months (Monticello et al., 1996).

Glutaraldehyde

A series of repeated-dose experiments with rats and mice exposed to glutaraldehyde has been summarized by NICNAS (1994). Among these, the lowest concentration producing lesions of the nasal cavity of rats was 1000 $\mu g/m^3$ (6 h/day, 5 days/week, for 13 weeks) (NTP, 1993). The most severe lesions occurred in the anterior portions of the nasal passages and involved both the respiratory and olfactory epithelium. Hyperplasia and squamous metaplasia were most commonly noted on the lateral wall of the nasal cavity and on the tips of the nasoturbinates. Lesions were most extensive in rats exposed to 4000 $\mu g/m^3$, but were also noted in the 1000 and 2000 $\mu g/m^3$ groups and in one male exposed to 500 $\mu g/m^3$. In another study in rats, no nasal lesions were observed at concentrations up to 776 $\mu g/m^3$ delivered for 14 weeks (Bushy Run, 1983).

Mice appeared to be more sensitive to glutaraldehyde inhalation in a 13-week study, with inflammation of the nasal cavity being observed in female mice even at the lowest concentration of 250 $\mu g/m^3$ and in male mice at 1000 $\mu g/m^3$. The species difference in sensitivity is probably due to the smaller airways of mice being more prone to blockage by debris (NTP, 1993). Histopathological lesions in the respiratory tract were most severe in mice in the 4000 µg/m³ group and consisted of minimal to mild squamous metaplasia of the laryngeal epithelium, suppurative inflammation in the anterior parts of the nasal cavity, and minimal squamous metaplasia on the tips of the nasoturbinates. Necrosis and inflammation were noted at lower concentrations, primarily in the anterior portion of the nasal passage.

In the NTP (1993) 13-week studies with glutaraldehyde, there were significant, exposure-related increases in ULLI in the squamous epithelium of the nasal vestibule and, to a lesser extent, the respiratory epithelium of the atrioturbinate of the dorsal meatus. The exposure-related increase in cell replication was generally greater in rats than in mice. Upon examining the results in individual mice, it was found that there was an increased rate of cell replication in the squamous epithelium of the nasal vestibule only of those mice in which there was also neutrophilic infiltration of the mucosa; however, the severity of the infiltrate did not correlate with the degree of cell proliferation. These observations were clearest at 13 weeks, particularly in female mice. In rats, in addition to increased replication in the squamous epithelium of the vestibule, there was an equally prominent increase in replication in the respiratory epithelium of the dorsal atrioturbinate, whereas in mice, the response in this area was weak.

D. Temporal association

Formaldehyde

A number of short-, medium-, and long-term studies of the effect of formaldehyde exposure on cell proliferation within the respiratory epithelium of rats have indicated a sustained increase in proliferation of nasal epithelial cells following exposure to concentrations greater than 2.4 mg/m³, irrespective of the exposure period. Cell proliferation was observed in rats exposed to formaldehyde for periods from as short as 3 days. In the ULLI study already described, the magnitude of increased cell proliferation generally decreased over time but remained significantly increased by approximately 2- to 10-fold over controls, for certain nasal locations, up to and including the 18-month observation period when this effect was last examined (Monticello et al., 1996).

Data relating to temporal associations for DPX are limited, as most formaldehyde inhalation studies of DPX formation are of short duration (i.e. exposure duration up to 1 day). Formaldehyde-induced DPX in the nasal epithelium of rats and rhesus monkeys was shown consistently in these studies (Casanova et al., 1991). However, a well conducted study investigating both acute and cumulative DPX yields in rats exposed to formaldehyde for about 12 weeks (Casanova et al., 1994) found that the acute DPX yield in the lateral meatus (a high tumour yield site) of previously exposed rats was about half that in naive rats at concentrations greater than 7.2 mg/m³, while there were no differences in the medial and posterior meatuses (low tumour yield sites). No significant accumulation of DPX occurred in previously exposed rats.

Regenerative cell proliferation following formaldehyde-induced cytotoxicity increases the number of DNA replications and thus increases the probability of DPX-initiated DNA replication errors, resulting in mutations. This hypothesis is supported by the observed inhibition of DNA replication in the rat nose at elevated concentrations (Heck & Casanova, 1995) and increased p53 expression in preneoplastic lesions (Wolf et al., 1995). In 5 of 11 squamous cell carcinomas from rats exposed to 18 mg/m^3 for up to 2 years, there were point mutations at the GC base pairs in the p53 complementary DNA (cDNA) sequence (Recio et al., 1992).

Glutaraldehyde

The study of cell replication in the 13-week rat and mouse inhalation studies with glutaraldehyde (NTP, 1993) showed that, in contrast to the results obtained for mice, the increased cell replication (ULLI) in the nasal vestibule of rats occurred early (within a few days) and either remained elevated or decreased slightly through the course of the study. Increases in ULLI in the nasal vestibule of mice tended to develop with time. In an inhalation study with mice (Zissu et al., 1994), the earliest lesions were observed in the respiratory epithelium of the septum and the naso- and maxilloturbinates after 4 days of exposure to 1.2 mg/m^3. Severe histopathological changes were still observed 2 weeks after the end of the exposure to 4.0 mg/m^3. No exposure-related histological abnormalities were detected in the trachea and lungs.

E. Strength, consistency, and specificity of association of tumour response with key events

Formaldehyde

There are extensive studies investigating formaldehyde-induced neoplasia. Available data revealed formaldehyde-induced DPX formation and increased epithelial cell proliferation within the upper respiratory tract in a range of species including rats and monkeys and a variety of rat and human cells in vitro. It was found that at similar levels of exposure, concentrations of DPX were approximately an order of magnitude lower in rhesus monkeys than in rats. Increased human epithelial cell proliferation following in situ exposure to formaldehyde was reported in a model system in which rat tracheae populated with human tracheobronchial epithelial cells were xenotransplanted into athymic mice.

There is good correlation between key events and regional tumour incidence and tumour sites. Cell proliferation, metaplasia, and increased DPX were seen in the regions of the nasal cavity where tumours have been observed. The highly non-linear dose–response relationships for DPX, cytotoxicity, cell proliferation, metaplasia, and tumours are consistent, with significant increases in metaplasia occurring at 2.4 mg/m^3 in one study and all end-points being observed at concentrations of greater than 4.8 mg/m^3. This is also in good correlation with the concentration at which mucociliary clearance is inhibited and glutathione-mediated metabolism is saturated—that is, 4.8 mg/m^3. The study by Morgan et al. (1986) examining effects of inhaled formaldehyde on the nasal mucociliary apparatus in male rats also included 18-h recovery groups following days 1, 9, and 14 of exposure to concentrations of 2.4 mg/m^3, 7.2 mg/m^3, and 18 mg/m^3. Inhibition of mucociliary clearance was progressively more extensive with increasing duration of exposure, but showed little or no evidence of recovery 18 h after cessation of exposure.

Mice appear to be less susceptible than rats to the development of nasal tumours following exposure to a given concentration of formaldehyde. However, it is well known that mice decrease their minute volume in response to inhalation of noxious chemicals (Brown et al., 1986, in CIIT, 1999).

Glutaraldehyde

In comparison with formaldehyde, the glutaraldehyde-induced lesions were located in a more anterior part of the nose, involving the squamous epithelium. Also, they were of a different character, with none of the focal hyperkeratosis and hyperplasia with cellular atypia and dysplasia found in animals receiving formaldehyde for 13 weeks (Monticello, 1990; Morgan & Monticello, 1990).

F. Biological plausibility and coherence

Formaldehyde

Evidence supporting the hypothesis that prolonged regenerative cell proliferation can be a causal mechanism in chemical carcinogenesis continues to accumulate (IPCS, 2002). This proposed MOA for formaldehyde-induced nasal tumours in animals exposed by inhalation is consistent with biological plausibility and the available data. Sustained increased cell proliferation has been observed in the nasal cavity in extensive short- and medium-term toxicity studies in rats and a few studies in other species. Histopathological effects in the nasal cavity (epithelial cell dysplasia and metaplasia) were consistent in a range of sub-chronic and chronic animal studies. It should be noted, however, that the respective roles of DPX, mutation, and cellular proliferation in the induction of nasal tumours in the rat have not been fully elucidated.

Glutaraldehyde

Effects of inhaled glutaraldehyde have not been as extensively studied as those of formaldehyde. In inhalation studies, glutaraldehyde did not induce nasal tumours in rats and mice. However, the same key events that are considered key events in the nasal carcino-genicity of formaldehyde—cytotoxicity and cell proliferation—have been demonstrated in rats and mice exposed to glutaraldehyde. This might appear to reduce the plausibility of these processes being important for formaldehyde.

G. Possible alternative modes of action

Formaldehyde

There is the possibility that mutagenicity could play a role in the development of formal-dehyde-induced tumours. Evaluation of the available data indicates that formaldehyde is genotoxic in vitro, but is generally not genotoxic in standard in vivo assays, although there are many studies demonstrating that it produces DPX.

Formaldehyde has been extensively studied for genotoxicity in vitro, with positive results in studies with bacterial and mammalian cells (Ames test, gene mutation), and produced DNA single-strand breaks and DPX (reviewed in IARC, 2005). In vivo, formaldehyde has repro-ducibly induced mutations in *Drosophila*, but there is no convincing evidence of its genotoxic activity in rodent bone marrow cell tests. There is limited evidence that formaldehyde exposure is associated with increased chromosomal aberration and micronucleus frequencies in human nasal and buccal cells and peripheral blood lymphocytes (reviewed in IARC, 2005; see Appendix).

It is unclear to what extent DPX contributes to the mutagenesis and carcinogenicity of formaldehyde (Recio, 1997; Merk & Speit, 1998; Speit et al., 2000; Liteplo & Meek, 2003). The presence of DPX has been considered mainly as an indicator of exposure, although some have also seen these lesions as premutagenic in character and therefore evidence of a direct genotoxic mechanism. DPX are, however, potentially damaging to the afflicted cell, and cell death is a likely outcome should they occur at high frequency. They also indicate that protein–protein cross-linkage (PPX) may occur, with potentially less serious effects for the cell. Should key proteins be involved in the PPX formation, this could have consequences on the regulatory machinery of the cell, including the regulation of differentiation. Such a change clearly occurs in the nasal epithelium of rats exposed to formaldehyde, since areas of metaplasia emerge. Neoplasia could be viewed as simply a different kind of metaplasia, unless there is compelling evidence for a genotoxic mode of action.

A different interpretation of the data has been offered by Gaylor et al. (2004), who analysed the concentration–response relationship for formaldehyde-induced cell proliferation in rats using statistical methods designed to identify J-shaped concentration curves. Cell proliferation data were used because there were insufficient quantal data on cancer incidence to perform the analysis. Their analysis supports the hypothesis that the threshold-type dose–response for nasal tumour incidence is the result of a minor genotoxicity at low dose that is superimposed by a J-shaped dose–response for cell proliferation at high cytotoxic dose levels (Lutz, 1998). At low doses, the effect of incremental DNA damage may be cancelled out by a reduction in cell proliferation; therefore, in spite of the apparent threshold, the data remain consistent with a genotoxic mechanism.

In rats exposed to formaldehyde, point mutations at GC base pairs in the cDNA sequence of the evolutionarily conserved regions II–V of the *p53* gene were found in 5 of 11 primary nasal squamous cell carcinomas (Recio et al., 1992). This observation may be interpreted to indicate genotoxic processes induced by formaldehyde in the carcinogenic process; however, the presence of specific mutations in the emergent tumour is not evidence that they were present in the early stages of neoplasia or that they were directly induced by the chemical. While there is the possibility of a direct mutagenic event occurring, it is also possible that these mutations arose indirectly of exposure as a result of functional changes in chromatin proteins induced by the chemical. At what stage in the life history of the tumour these observed mutations occurred is also open to speculation: they are relatively common events, it is clear, but it is also clear that they are not essential events (since they do not occur in all tumours that are apparently of the same type). The occurrence of these mutations indicates that a genotoxic mechanism has not been excluded, but this evidence does not necessarily support one.

Specific changes in gene expression have also been observed in vivo. The results indicated that exposure to formaldehyde can cause alteration in the expression levels of genes involved in several functional categories, including xenobiotic metabolism, cell cycle regulation, DNA synthesis and repair, oncogenes, and apoptosis (Hester et al., 2003). It is not clear at present how specific these changes are to formaldehyde or what their role is, if any, in carcinogenicity.

Glutaraldehyde

Glutaraldehyde has been less extensively tested than formaldehyde for genotoxicity in vitro and in vivo. It produces weak and inconsistent positive findings in tests in vitro and is not active in the vast majority of in vivo studies. The genetic toxicity of glutaraldehyde has been recently reviewed (Zeiger et al., 2005).

Glutaraldehyde induced DNA repair systems in bacterial cells and was a weak mutagen in *Salmonella* and *Escherichia coli*. Unscheduled DNA synthesis (UDS), DPX, and double-strand breaks were seen in human cell lines, but not in primary rat cells. There were weak and inconsistent responses in chromosomal aberration and sister chromatid exchange (SCE) studies with mammalian cells, and glutaraldehyde did not induce transformation in cultured Syrian hamster embryo (SHE) cells.

In vivo, glutaraldehyde induced S-phase DNA synthesis in nasal cells in rats and mice following direct nasal administration. Glutaraldehyde did not produce DNA damage in rat liver or cross-links in rat testes DNA or sperm cells. Tests for induction of chromosomal aberration in bone marrow cells in rats and mice were generally negative. Glutaraldehyde did not induce micronuclei in bone marrow cells or dominant lethal mutations in mice. Thus, glutaraldehyde does possess genotoxic potential, and, although the database is not as extensive as it is for formaldehyde, it might be anticipated that site of contact genotoxicity would occur. Consequently, if genotoxicity is a major carcinogenic MOA for formaldehyde, it remains to be explained why glutaraldehyde is not active.

H. Uncertainties, inconsistencies, and data gaps

Formaldehyde

In most of the cancer bioassays for formaldehyde, data on intermediate end-points such as proliferative response as a measure of cytotoxicity and DPX are limited. Consequently, direct comparison of the incidence of intermediate lesions and tumours is restricted. Additionally, information on a direct relationship between DPX and mutation induction and the probability of converting a DPX into a mutation is desirable, while the mode by which regenerative cell proliferation is involved in the production of mutations required for tumour development needs to be determined.

Studies on the *hprt* mutation spectrum in formaldehyde-exposed human cells revealed that 50% of the mutations are deletions, whereas 50% are due to point mutation at the A:T base pair (Crosby et al., 1988; Liber et al., 1989). The finding of deletions as part of the formaldehyde mutation spectrum may explain the homozygous nature of base pair mutations observed in *p53* in formaldehyde-induced squamous cell carcinomas. However, there is an inconsistency with regard to the base pair that is mutated. It was found to be A:T in *hprt* in human and mammalian cell lines and G:C at *p53* in formaldehyde-induced squamous cell carcinomas (Recio, 1997). It is possible that, although mutations are induced by formaldehyde in vitro, these types of mutation may not be fundamental to its carcinogenicity.

86

Glutaraldehyde

Glutaraldehyde is clearly much more cytotoxic than formaldehyde, perhaps because it is a bifunctional alkylating agent. Intranasal instillation studies have demonstrated that, on a molar basis, glutaraldehyde is 10- to 20-fold more toxic than formaldehyde when delivered to the nasal mucosa as a single treatment in aqueous solution (St. Clair et al., 1990). Comparison of results from a 13-week inhalation study of glutaraldehyde (NTP, 1993) with similar inhalation studies with formaldehyde (Heck et al., 1990; Monticello, 1990; Monticello et al., 1991) shows that glutaraldehyde is about 20-fold more toxic than formaldehyde by this route also. Pulmonary damage and mortality occur at much higher glutaraldehyde concentrations. Cytotoxicity is manifest closer to the external nares in the case of inhaled glutaraldehyde, so the tissue primarily affected is not the same as in the case of inhaled formaldehyde. This difference in the site of toxic action may be particularly important because, if the only difference was toxic potency, then glutaraldehyde would be expected to produce effects similar to those of formaldehyde, although only at lower doses.

I. Assessment of postulated mode of action

Formaldehyde

From a weight-of-evidence point of view, the hypothesized MOA for formaldehyde-induced nasal tumours satisfies several criteria, including consistency, concordance of dose–response relationships across all key events, and biological plausibility and coherence of the database. Given the extensive experimental data that address and are consistent with the proposed MOA of formaldehyde in the induction of tumours in the nasal cavity, a high degree of confidence may be ascribed to it.

Glutaraldehyde

The key events of cytotoxicity, cell proliferation, and DPX formation (in vitro) have been demonstrated with exposure to glutaraldehyde. However, glutaraldehyde has not produced nasal tumours in rats and mice. Therefore, if the proposed MOA for formaldehyde is to be maintained, an explanation for this discrepancy is necessary. A reason for the difference has not been identified, but a hypothesis can be proposed. The dialdehyde function of glutaraldehyde is an important factor that may inhibit the macromolecules with which it reacts from further reaction within the cellular environment. Should these macromolecules be proteins involved in the maintenance of survival, then their immobility perhaps more likely leads to cell death than to a change in differentiation state. This immobilization of macromolecules by glutaraldehyde is the property that makes it a better fixative for high-resolution microscopy (e.g. electron microscopy) than formaldehyde. It almost certainly contributes to the very much higher toxicity of the dialdehyde. The monoaldehyde function of formaldehyde also causes cellular damage, but a proportion of proteins involved in cellular differentiation may be able to continue in that role, although with an altered outcome that may be the beginning of a path to neoplasia. If, on the other hand, these aldehydes react with nucleic acids (the evidence for glutaraldehyde reacting in this way is not substantial), then the repair of the alkylated nucleotides may be more difficult or even impossible in the case of glutaraldehyde, whereas repair does occur following formaldehyde interaction with DNA. Thus, irrespective of whether the mode of formaldehyde action in carcinogenicity is as proposed or is primarily due to genetic toxicity, the different response to glutaraldehyde exposure can be explained.

2. CAN HUMAN RELEVANCE OF THE MOA BE EXCLUDED ON THE BASIS OF FUNDAMENTAL, QUALITATIVE DIFFERENCES IN KEY EVENTS BETWEEN EXPERIMENTAL ANIMALS AND HUMANS?

A. Formaldehyde

In rhesus monkeys exposed to formaldehyde at 7.2 mg/m^3 for between 1 and 6 weeks, formaldehyde-induced lesions were associated with increases in cell proliferation rates of up to 18-fold over controls and remained significantly elevated after 6 weeks of exposure. Histological lesions and increases in cell proliferation were most extensive in the nasal passages and were minimal in the lower airways, whereas the maxillary sinuses showed no evidence of a response to formaldehyde exposure. Based on the extent of lesions and cell proliferation data, it appeared that rhesus monkeys are more sensitive than rats to the acute and subacute effects of formaldehyde at 7.2 mg/m^3 (Monticello et al., 1989). The absence of response in the maxillary sinuses in rhesus monkeys is an observation deserving special attention in the design of epidemiological studies (or, perhaps, in the reporting of tumour sites). Most epidemiological studies of sinonasal cancer have not distinguished tumours arising in the nose from those developing in the nasal sinuses. Thus, the risk for nasal cancer specifically would tend to be diluted if there was no corresponding risk for cancer in the sinuses and could go undetected through lack of statistical power.

Many epidemiological studies have investigated formaldehyde exposure and cancer of the respiratory tract. The strongest evidence of an association has been observed for nasopharyngeal cancers. A statistically significant excess of deaths from nasopharyngeal cancer has been observed in the largest cohort study of industrial workers (Hauptmann et al., 2004), with statistically significant exposure–response relationships for peak and cumulative exposure. An excess of deaths from nasopharyngeal cancer was observed in a proportionate mortality analysis of the largest cohort of embalmers in the United States (Hayes et al., 1990). An excess of cases of nasopharyngeal cancer was observed in a Danish study of proportionate cancer incidence among workers at companies that manufactured or used formaldehyde (Hansen & Olsen, 1995). Other cohort studies reported fewer cases of nasopharyngeal cancer than expected (Walrath & Fraumeni, 1983; Coggon et al., 2003; Pinkerton et al., 2004). Of seven case–control studies of nasopharyngeal cancer, five found elevations of risk for exposure to formaldehyde.

Several case–control studies have investigated the association between exposure to formaldehyde and sinonasal cancer. A pooled analysis of 12 studies showed an increased risk of adenocarcinoma in men and women thought never to have been exposed to wood dust or leather dust, with an exposure–response trend for an index of cumulative exposure (Luce et al., 2002). One other case–control study (Olsen & Asnaes, 1986) and a proportionate incidence study (Hansen & Olsen, 1995) showed an increased risk of sinonasal cancer, particularly squamous cell carcinoma. However, the three most informative cohort studies of industrial workers showed no excesses of sinonasal cancer (Coggon et al., 2003; Hauptmann et al., 2004; Pinkerton et al., 2004).

In evaluating this body of evidence, the International Agency for Research on Cancer (IARC) concluded that there was sufficient epidemiological evidence that formaldehyde causes nasopharyngeal cancer in humans; only limited epidemiological evidence that formaldehyde causes sinonasal cancer in humans; and strong but not sufficient evidence for a causal association between leukaemia and occupational exposure to formaldehyde (Cogliano et al., 2005).

There are no publications describing DPX in nasal cells from formaldehyde-exposed personnel. Assessment of DPX in peripheral lymphocytes from formaldehyde-exposed workers demonstrated an association with overall exposure (Shaham et al., 2003). The single DPX study involved 399 workers from 14 hospital pathology departments, and formaldehyde exposure categories were low-level (mean 0.5 mg/m^3, range 0.05–0.8 mg/m^3) and high-level (mean 2.7 mg/m^3, range 0.86–6.7 mg/m^3). Adjusted mean DPX were significantly higher in the exposed groups. There appear to be some doubts regarding the sensitivity and reproducibility of the physical separation method used in this study (Heck & Casanova, 2004).

Some studies have investigated the histological changes within the nasal epithelium of workers occupationally exposed to formaldehyde; however, the extent to which nasal epithelial cell regenerative proliferation occurs is unresolved because the results are mixed and there was co-exposure to wood dust in some studies (Berke, 1987; Edling et al., 1988; Holmström et al., 1989; Boysen et al., 1990; Ballarin et al., 1992).

Mucociliary clearance in the anterior portion of the nasal cavity was reduced following exposure of volunteers to formaldehyde at 0.30 mg/m^3 (Andersen & Mølhave, 1983).

The concordance of animal and human key events for formaldehyde is summarized in Table 3.

Table 3. Formaldehyde concordance table.

Key event	Evidence in animals	Evidence in humans
Cytotoxicity	Positive in vivo (target cells)	Plausible
Proliferation	Positive in vivo (target cells)	Plausible (some evidence but confounded by co-exposure)
Genotoxicity	DPX (target cells in vivo)	DPX (non-target cells, i.e. lymphocytes)
Mutations	Positive in vitro; unconvincing in vivo	Positive (? cells)
Nasal tumours	Positive (mainly anterior lateral meatus)	Positive (nasopharyngeal) ? (sinonasal)

B. Glutaraldehyde

There are few epidemiological studies for exposure to glutaraldehyde and human cancer. No increase in the number of cancer deaths was observed among 186 male glutaraldehyde production workers. The average time since first exposure to glutaraldehyde was 20.6 years, and the period of exposure was 3–7 years. During periods of monitoring exposure, glutaraldehyde concentrations in air ranged from 0.04 to 1.4 mg/m^3 (NICNAS, 1994). Studies of embalmers, pathologists, and members of the American Association of Anatomists for possible effects of glutaraldehyde have all shown increases in risk of cancer; however, all of these groups were also exposed to formaldehyde (Walrath & Fraumeni, 1983; Consensus Workshop on Formaldehyde, 1984; Stroup et al., 1986).

There are no studies examining glutaraldehyde exposure and DPX formation, cytotoxicity, and cell proliferation in human nasal tissues.

The concordance of animal and human key events for glutaraldehyde is summarized in Table 4.

Table 4. Glutaraldehyde concordance table.

Key event	Evidence in animals	Evidence in humans
Cytotoxicity	Positive	Plausible
Proliferation	Positive in vivo	Plausible
Genotoxicity	DPX in vitro	Unknown
Mutations	Positive in vitro	Unknown
Nasal tumours	Negative (no evidence at any site)	Unknown

3. CAN HUMAN RELEVANCE OF THE MOA BE EXCLUDED ON THE BASIS OF QUANTITATIVE DIFFERENCES IN EITHER KINETIC OR DYNAMIC FACTORS BETWEEN EXPERIMENTAL ANIMALS AND HUMANS?

A. Formaldehyde

Quantitative differences between experimental animals and humans for the postulated MOA will be a function of the concentration of formaldehyde at the target tissue. It is formaldehyde per se, and not its metabolites, that causes cytotoxicity. Exogenous inhaled formaldehyde is rapidly metabolized upon absorption, to formate, by a number of widely distributed cellular enzymes, particularly formaldehyde dehydrogenase. In addition to this efficient metabolic detoxification mechanism, the mucociliary apparatus provides protection of the underlying epithelium from gases and vapours. Thus, in order to attain free formaldehyde concentrations that may be cytotoxic to the target tissue, relatively high concentrations of formaldehyde vapour must be delivered to the target site to overcome these protective mechanisms. Mechanistic events of clear significance for carcinogenicity occur at dose levels where formaldehyde detoxification mechanisms are saturated in rats (Casanova & Heck, 1987).

It is critical to take dosimetry into consideration when considering quantitative species differences for formaldehyde-induced toxicity in the respiratory tract. Inhaled formaldehyde is predominantly deposited and readily absorbed in the regions of the upper respiratory tract with which it comes into initial contact, owing to its high reactivity with biological macromolecules (Heck et al., 1983; Swenberg et al., 1983). A complex relationship between nasal anatomy, ventilation, and breathing patterns (nasal or oronasal) determines where in the upper respiratory tract formaldehyde absorption occurs in species. In rodents, which are obligate nasal breathers, deposition and absorption occur primarily in the nasal passage. In contrast, primates are oronasal breathers; although absorption and deposition are likely to occur primarily in the oral mucosa and nasal passages, they can also occur in the trachea and bronchus (Monticello et al., 1991). This hypothesis is supported by effects (histopathological changes, increased epithelial cell proliferation, and DPX formation) being observed farther along within the upper respiratory tract in monkeys.

Species differences in dosimetry have been taken into account in a two-stage clonal growth model that has been developed to predict the nasal carcinogenic risk of formaldehyde in humans (Conolly et al., 2004). The model also incorporates data on normal growth curves for rats and humans, cell cycle times, and cells at risk in the different regions of the respiratory tract.

Mice are better able to reduce both their respiratory rate and tidal volume upon repeated exposures; therefore, mice have less formaldehyde available for deposition than rats, resulting in less tissue damage and a lower rate of cell turnover in the nasal epithelium (Chang et al., 1981, 1983). These are characteristics that may help explain the lack of neoplastic response in the nose of mice.

Although there are likely to be quantitative differences between animal species and humans due to differences in dosimetry in the respiratory tract, there do not appear to be fundamental differences that would indicate that the proposed MOA does not occur in humans.

B. Glutaraldehyde

Much less is known of the kinetics of glutaraldehyde in experimental animals compared with formaldehyde. Inhalation studies do not appear to have been conducted. The terminal half-lives for elimination are long for both intravenous injection (rat 10 h, rabbit 15–30 h) and dermal application (rat 40–110 h, rabbit 20–100 h), probably due to the binding of glutaraldehyde to protein and the slow excretion of metabolites. The metabolites have not been identified, but it has been proposed that the metabolism of glutaraldehyde probably involves initial oxidation to the corresponding carboxylic acids by aldehyde dehydrogenase. The glutaric acid formed by oxidation is probably further metabolized by reaction with coenzyme A (CoA) to give glutaryl CoA, which is then oxidized by glutaryl CoA dehydrogenase to glutaconyl CoA, leading to its eventual degradation to carbon dioxide via acetate (Beauchamp et al., 1992; NTP, 1993; NICNAS, 1994; Ballantyne, 1995).

Glutaraldehyde reacts readily with proteins as a cross-linking agent, mainly between amino groups. The reaction is rapid and pH dependent (rate increases at pH >9), to give Schiff bases. Further reaction occurs to give a number of complex reaction products, with the mechanism of the cross-linking process not yet fully understood.

Little information is available on the interaction between glutaraldehyde and DNA, but it has been reported (Hopwood, 1975) that glutaraldehyde reacts with DNA only at >60 °C (summarized by NICNAS, 1994), and there are data implying that there is no reaction under physiological conditions (Sewell et al., 1984; Douglas & Rogers, 1998; Vock et al., 1999).

4. STATEMENT OF CONFIDENCE, ANALYSIS, AND IMPLICATION

A. Formaldehyde

Sustained cytotoxicity and cell proliferation are key events in the proposed MOA for the induction of several types of animal tumours. There are substantial data to support this postulated MOA for formaldehyde-induced nasal tumours in rats. Cytotoxicity, DPX formation, nasal epithelial cell regenerative proliferation, squamous metaplasia, and inflammation have been measured in rat studies and are site-specific, highly non-linear concentration–response processes in concordance with the incidence of nasal tumours.

Based on the weight of evidence, it is likely that the MOA is relevant to humans, at least qualitatively. Increased cell proliferation and DPX formation within epithelia of the upper respiratory tract have been observed in monkeys exposed to formaldehyde vapour. Increased human epithelial cell proliferation following in situ exposure to formaldehyde has also been observed in a model system in which rat tracheae populated with human tracheobronchial epithelial cells were xenotransplanted into athymic mice. Limited evidence on histo-pathological lesions in the nose of humans exposed primarily to formaldehyde in the occupational environment is consistent with a qualitatively similar response of the upper respiratory tract in experimental animals. In addition, several epidemiological studies have indicated an increased risk of nasal cancers with formaldehyde exposure.

Therefore, the MOA is considered relevant to humans, and animal nasal tumour and other supporting data should be taken forward to evaluate human risk. This process would include consideration of the data suggesting that formaldehyde induces tumours in a non-linear, dose-dependent manner. There may also be quantitative differences in response between species for the proposed MOA due to differences in dosimetry.

B. Glutaraldehyde

The epidemiological studies for glutaraldehyde are very limited and do not show an association with nasal tumours. In animal studies, glutaraldehyde has been shown to cause cytotoxicity, cell proliferation, and DPX production, but not nasal tumours, in inhalation studies in rats and mice. The fact that glutaraldehyde is clearly more toxic than formaldehyde should not constitute a reason for the difference in carcinogenic potential. Although, dose for dose, glutaraldehyde exposure may tend to result in more cell death than formaldehyde exposure, if glutaraldehyde is a carcinogen, this should be demonstrable at doses lower than those used for formaldehyde.

The MOA postulated for formaldehyde—that is, sustained cytotoxicity and cell proliferation—would appear to be relevant to glutaraldehyde, but tumour formation has not been demonstrated. It has been tentatively suggested here that the difference in pathological responses to these aldehydes is due to formaldehyde being a monoaldehyde whereas glutar-aldehyde is a dialdehyde. This difference may result in a different form of cross-linking so that glutaraldehyde cross-link products are neither likely to retain any biological function nor likely to be repairable. The case-study highlights the difficulties in applying the HRF when the animal tumour data are inadequate.

REFERENCES

Andersen I, Mølhave L (1983) Controlled human studies with formaldehyde. In: Gibson JE, ed. *Formaldehyde toxicity*. Washington, DC, Hemisphere Publishing, pp. 155–165.

Ballantyne B (1995) *Toxicology of glutaraldehyde: Review of studies and human health effects*. Bound Brook, NJ, Union Carbide Corporation.

Ballarin C, Sarto F, Giacomelli L, Bartolucci GB, Clonfero E (1992) Micronucleated cells in nasal mucosa of formaldehyde-exposed workers. *Mutation Research*, **280**:1–7.

Beauchamp ROJ, St Clair MB, Fennell TR, Clarke DO, Morgan KT, Kari FW (1992) A critical review of the toxicology of glutaraldehyde. *Critical Reviews in Toxicology*, **22**:143–174.

Berke JH (1987) Cytologic examination of the nasal mucosa in formaldehyde-exposed workers. *Journal of Occupational Medicine*, **29**:681–684.

Boysen M, Zadig E, Digernes V, Abeler V, Reith A (1990) Nasal mucosa in workers exposed to formaldehyde: A pilot study. *British Journal of Industrial Medicine*, **47**:116–121.

Burgaz S, Cakmak G, Erdem O, Yilmaz M, Karakaya AE (2001) Micronuclei frequencies in exfoliated nasal mucosa cells from pathology and anatomy laboratory workers exposed to formaldehyde. *Neoplasma*, **48**:144–147.

Burgaz S, Erdem O, Cakmak G, Erdem N, Karakaya A, Karakaya AE (2002) Cytogenetic analysis of buccal cells from shoe-workers and pathology and anatomy laboratory workers exposed to *n*-hexane, toluene, methyl ethyl ketone and formaldehyde. *Biomarkers*, **7**:151–161.

Bushy Run (1983) *Glutaraldehyde vapour subchronic inhalation study on rats*. Export, PA, Bushy Run Research Center (Project Report 46-101).

Casanova M, Heck Hd'A (1987) Further studies of the metabolic incorporation and covalent binding of inhaled [^{3}H]- and [^{14}C]formaldehyde in Fischer-344 rats: Effects of glutathione depletion. *Toxicology and Applied Pharmacology*, **89**:105–121.

Casanova M, Heck Hd'A, Everitt JI, Harrington WW Jr, Popp JA (1988) Formaldehyde concentrations in the blood of rhesus monkeys after inhalation exposure. *Food and Chemical Toxicology*, **26**:715–716.

Casanova M, Deyo DF, Heck Hd'A (1989) Covalent binding of inhaled formaldehyde to DNA in the nasal mucosa of Fischer 344 rats: Analysis of formaldehyde and DNA by high-performance liquid chromatography and provisional pharmacokinetic interpretation. *Fundamental and Applied Toxicology*, **12**:397–417.

Casanova M, Morgan KT, Steinhagen WH, Everitt JI, Popp JA, Heck Hd'A (1991) Covalent binding of inhaled formaldehyde to DNA in the respiratory tract of rhesus monkeys: Pharmacokinetics, rat-to-monkey interspecies scaling, and extrapolation to man. *Fundamental and Applied Toxicology*, **17**:409–428.

Casanova M, Morgan KT, Gross EA, Moss OR, Heck Hd'A (1994) DNA–protein cross-links and cell replication at specific sites in the nose of F344 rats exposed subchronically to formaldehyde. *Fundamental and Applied Toxicology*, **23**:525–536.

Casanova-Schmitz M, Starr TB, Heck H (1984) Differentiation between metabolic incorporation and covalent binding in the labeling of macromolecules in the rat nasal mucosa and bone marrow by inhaled [^{14}C]- and [^{3}H]formaldehyde. *Toxicology and Applied Pharmacology*, **76**:26–44.

Chang JCF, Steinhagen WH, Barrow CS (1981) Effects of single or repeated formaldehyde exposures on minute volume of B6C3F1 mice and F344 rats. *Toxicology and Applied Pharmacology*, **61**:451–459.

Chang JCF, Gross EA, Swenberg JA, Barrow CS (1983) Nasal cavity deposition, histopathology and cell proliferation after single or repeated formaldehyde exposures in B6C3F1 mice and F-344 rats. *Toxicology and Applied Pharmacology*, **68**:161–176.

CIIT (1999) *Formaldehyde: Hazard characterization and dose–response assessment for carcinogenicity by the route of inhalation*, rev. ed. Research Triangle Park, NC, Chemical Industry Institute of Toxicology.

Coggon D, Harris EC, Poole J, Palmer KT (2003) Extended follow-up of a cohort of British chemical workers exposed to formaldehyde. *Journal of the National Cancer Institute*, **21**:1608–1614.

Cogliano VJ, Grosse Y, Baan RA, Straif K, Secretan MB, El Ghissassi F (2005) Meeting report: Summary of IARC Monographs on formaldehyde, 2-butoxyethanol and 1-*tert*-butoxy-2-propanol. *Environmental Health Perspectives*, **113**(9):1205–1208.

Conolly RB, Kimbell JS, Janszen D, Schlosser PM, Kalisak D, Preston J, Miller FJ (2004) Human respiratory tract cancer risks of inhaled formaldehyde: Dose–response predictions derived from biologically-motivated computational modeling of a combined rodent and human dataset. *Toxicological Sciences*, **82**:279–296.

Consensus Workshop on Formaldehyde (1984) Report on the consensus workshop on formaldehyde. *Environmental Health Perspectives*, **58**:323–381.

Crosby RM, Richardson KK, Craft TR, Benforado KB, Liber HL, Skopek TR (1988) Molecular analysis of formaldehyde-induced mutations in human lymphoblasts and *E. coli*. *Environmental and Molecular Mutagenesis*, **12**:155–166.

Dalbey WE (1982) Formaldehyde and tumors in hamster respiratory tract. *Toxicology*, **24**:9–14.

Douglas MP, Rogers SO (1998) DNA damage caused by common cytological fixatives. *Mutation Research*, **401**:77–88.

Edling C, Hellquist H, Ödkvist L (1988) Occupational exposure to formaldehyde and histopathological changes in the nasal mucosa. *British Journal of Industrial Medicine*, **45**:761–765.

Feron VJ, Bruyntes JP, Woutersen RA, Immel HR, Appelman LM (1988) Nasal tumours in rats after short-term exposure to a cytotoxic concentration of formaldehyde. *Cancer Letters*, **39**:101–111.

Feron VJ, Til HP, Woutersen RA (1990) Letter to the editor. *Toxicology and Industrial Health*, **6**:637–639.

Gaylor DW, Lutz WK, Connolly RB (2004) Statistical analysis of nonmonotonic dose–response relationships: Research design and analysis of nasal cell proliferation in rats exposed to formaldehyde. *Toxicological Sciences*, **77**:158–164.

Gross EA, Mellick PW, Kari FW, Miller FJ, Morgan KT (1994) Histopathology and cell replication responses in the respiratory tract of rats and mice exposed by inhalation to glutaraldehyde for up to 13 weeks. *Fundamental and Applied Toxicology*, **23**:348–362.

Hansen J, Olsen JH (1995) Formaldehyde and cancer morbidity among male employees in Denmark. *Cancer Causes and Control*, **6**:354–360.

Hardman JG, Limbird LE, Gilman AG, eds (2001) *Goodman & Gilman's The pharmacological basis of therapeutics*, 10th ed. The McGraw-Hill Companies, Inc., 2025 pp.

Hauptmann A, Lubin JH, Stewart PA, Hayes RB, Blair A (2004). Mortality from solid cancers among workers in formaldehyde industries. *American Journal of Epidemiology*, **159**:1117–1130.

Hayes RB, Blair A, Stewart PA, Herrick RF, Mahar H (1990) Mortality of U.S. embalmers and funeral directors. *American Journal of Industrial Medicine*, **18**:641–652.

He J-L, Jin L-F, Jin H-Y (1998) Detection of cytogenetic effects in peripheral lymphocytes of students exposed to formaldehyde with cytokinesis-blocked micronucleus assay. *Biomedical and Environmental Sciences*, **11**:87–92.

Heck H, Casanova M (1995). Nasal dosimetry of formaldehyde: Modelling site specificity and the effects of pre-exposure. In: Miller JF, ed. *Nasal toxicity and dosimetry of inhaled xenobiotics: Implications for human health*. Washington, DC, Taylor & Francis, pp. 159–175.

Heck H, Casanova M (2004) The implausibility of leukemia induction by formaldehyde: A critical review of the biological evidence on distant-site toxicity. *Regulatory Toxicology and Pharmacology*, **40**:92–106.

Heck Hd'A, White EL, Casanova-Schmitz M (1982) Determination of formaldehyde in biological tissues by gas chromatography/mass spectrometry. *Biomedical Mass Spectrometry*, **9**:347–353.

Heck Hd'A, Chin TY, Schmitz MC (1983) Distribution of [^{14}C]formaldehyde in rats after inhalation exposure. In: Gibson JE, ed. *Formaldehyde toxicity*. Washington, DC, Hemisphere Publishing, pp. 26–37.

Heck Hd'A, Casanova-Schmitz M, Dodd PB, Schachter EN, Witek TJ, Tosun T (1985) Formaldehyde (CH_2O) concentrations in the blood of humans and Fischer-344 rats exposed to CH_2O under controlled conditions. *American Industrial Hygiene Association Journal*, **46**:1–3.

Heck Hd'A, Casanova M, Starr TB (1990) Formaldehyde toxicity—new understanding. *Critical Reviews in Toxicology*, **20**:397–426.

Hedberg JJ, Strömberg P, Höög JO (1998) An attempt to transform class characteristics within the alcohol dehydrogenase family. *FEBS Letters*, **436**:67–70.

Hester SD, Benavides GB, Yoon L, Morgan KT, Zou F, Barry W, Wolf DC (2003) Formaldehyde-induced gene expression in F344 rat nasal respiratory epithelium. *Toxicology*, **187**:13–24.

Holmquist B, Vallee BL (1991) Human liver class III alcohol and glutathione dependent formaldehyde dehydrogenase are the same enzyme. *Biochemical and Biophysical Research Communications*, **178**:1371–1377.

Holmström M, Wilhelmsson B, Hellquist H, Rosén G (1989) Histological changes in the nasal mucosa in persons occupationally exposed to formaldehyde alone and in combination with wood dust. *Acta Oto-laryngologica*, **107**:120–129.

Hopwood D (1975) The reactions of glutaraldehyde with nucleic acids. *Journal of Histochemistry*, **7**:267–276.

Horton AW, Tye R, Stemmer KL (1963) Experimental carcinogenesis of the lung. Inhalation of gaseous formaldehyde or an aerosol of coal tar by C3H mice. *Journal of the National Cancer Institute*, **30**:31–43.

IARC (2005) *Formaldehyde, 2-butoxyethanol and 1-tert-butoxypropan-2-ol*. Lyon, International Agency for Research on Cancer, 478 pp. (IARC Monographs on the Evaluation of Carcinogenic Risks to Humans, Vol. 88).

IPCS (2002) *Formaldehyde*. Geneva, World Health Organization, International Programme on Chemical Safety (Concise International Chemical Assessment Document No. 40).

Kamata E, Nakadate E, Uchida O, Ogawa Y, Suzuki S, Kaneko T, Saito M, Kurokawa Y (1997) Results of a 28-month chronic inhalation toxicity study of formaldehyde in male Fischer-344 rats. *Journal of Toxicological Sciences*, **22**:239–254.

Kerns WD, Pavkov KL, Donofrio DJ, Gralla EJ, Swenberg JA (1983a) Carcinogenicity of formaldehyde in rats and mice after long-term inhalation exposure. *Cancer Research*, **43**:4382–4392.

Kerns WD, Donofrio DJ, Pavkov KL (1983b) The chronic effects of formaldehyde inhalation in rats and mice: A preliminary report. In: Gibson JE, ed. *Formaldehyde toxicity*. Washington, DC, Hemisphere Publishing, pp. 111–131.

Kimbell JS, Gross EA, Richardson RB, Conolly RB, Morgan KT (1997) Correlation of regional formaldehyde flux predictions with the distribution of formaldehyde-induced squamous metaplasia in F344 rat nasal passages. *Mutation Research*, **380**:143–154.

Koivusalo M, Baumann M, Uotila L (1989) Evidence for the identity of glutathione-dependent formaldehyde dehydrogenase and class III alcohol dehydrogenase. *FEBS Letters*, **257**:105–109.

Liber HL, Benforado K, Crosby RM, Simpson D, Skopek TR (1989) Formaldehyde-induced and spontaneous alterations in human *hprt* DNA sequence and mRNA expression. *Mutation Research*, **226**:31–37.

Liteplo RG, Meek ME (2003) Inhaled formaldehyde: Exposure estimation, hazard characterization, and exposure–response analysis. *Journal of Toxicology and Environmental Health*, **B6**:85–114.

Luce D, Leclerc A, Begin D, Demers PA, Gerin M, Orlowski E, Kogevinas M, Belli S, Bugel I, Bolm-Audorff U, Brinton LA, Comba P, Hardell L, Hayes RB, Magnani C, Merler E, Preston-Martin S, Vaughan TL, Zheng W, Boffetta P (2002) Sinonasal cancer and occupational exposures: A pooled analysis of 12 case–control studies. *Cancer Causes and Control*, **13**:147–157.

Lutz WK (1998) Dose–response relationships in chemical carcinogenesis: Superposition of different mechanisms of action, resulting in linear–nonlinear curves, practical thresholds, J-shapes. *Mutation Research*, **405**:117–124.

Maronpot RR, Miller RA, Clarke WJ, Westerberg RB, Decker JR, Moss OR (1986) Toxicity of formaldehyde vapor in B6C3F1 mice exposed for 13 weeks. *Toxicology*, **41**:253–266.

Merk O, Speit G (1998) Significance of formaldehyde-induced DNA–protein crosslinks for mutagenesis. *Environmental and Molecular Mutagenesis*, **32**:260–268.

Monticello TM (1990) *Formaldehyde induced pathology and cell proliferation: A thesis.* Durham, NC, Duke University.

Monticello TM, Morgan KT (1994) Cell proliferation and formaldehyde-induced respiratory carcinogenesis. *Risk Analysis*, **14**:313–319.

Monticello TM, Morgan KT, Everitt JI, Popp JA (1989) Effects of formaldehyde gas on the respiratory tract of rhesus monkeys. Pathology and cell proliferation. *American Journal of Pathology*, **134**:515–527.

Monticello TM, Miller FJ, Morgan KT (1991) Regional increases in rat nasal epithelial cell proliferation following acute and subacute inhalation of formaldehyde. *Toxicology and Applied Pharmacology*, **111**:409–421.

Monticello TM, Swenberg JA, Gross EA, Leiniger JR, Kimbell JS, Seilkop S, Starr TB, Gibson JE, Morgan KT (1996) Correlation of regional and nonlinear formaldehyde-induced nasal cancer with proliferating populations of cells. *Cancer Research*, **56**:1012–1022.

Morgan KT, Monticello TM (1990) Formaldehyde toxicity: Respiratory epithelial injury and repair. In: Thomassen DG, Nettesheim P, eds. *Biology, toxicology, and carcinogenesis of the respiratory epithelium.* Washington, DC, Hemisphere Publishing, pp. 155–171.

Morgan KT, Jiang X-Z, Starr TB, Kerns WD (1986) More precise localization of nasal tumors associated with chronic exposure of F-344 rats to formaldehyde gas. *Toxicology and Applied Pharmacology*, **82**:264–271.

NICNAS (1994) *Glutaraldehyde. Full public report.* Canberra, Australian Government Publishing Service, National Industrial Chemicals Notification and Assessment Scheme, July (Priority Existing Chemical No. 3).

NTP (1993) *NTP technical report on toxicity studies on glutaraldehyde (CAS No. 111-30-8) administered by inhalation to F344/N rats and B6C3F1 mice.* Research Triangle Park, NC, National Institutes of Health, National Toxicology Program (NTP Toxicity Report No. 25; NIH Publication No. 93-3348).

NTP (1999) *Toxicology and carcinogenesis studies of glutaraldehyde (CAS No. 111-30-8) in F344/N rats and B6C3F1 mice (inhalation studies).* Research Triangle Park, NC, National Institutes of Health, National Toxicology Program (NTP Technical Report Series No. 490; NIH Publication No. 99-3980).

Olsen JH, Asnaes S (1986) Formaldehyde and the risk of squamous cell carcinoma of the sinonasal cavities. *British Journal of Industrial Medicine*, **43**:769–774.

Pinkerton L, Hein M, Stayner L (2004). Mortality among a cohort of garment workers exposed to formaldehyde: An update. *Occupational and Environmental Medicine*, **61**:193–200.

Recio L (1997) Oncogene and tumor suppressor gene alterations in nasal tumors. *Mutation Research*, **380**:27–31.

Recio L, Sisk S, Pluta L, Bermudez E, Gross EA, Chen Z, Morgan K, Walker C (1992) *p53* mutations in formaldehyde-induced nasal squamous cell carcinomas in rats. *Cancer Research*, **52**:6113–6116.

Rietbrock N (1965) [Formaldehyde oxidation in the rat.] *Naunyn-Schmiedebergs Archiv für experimentelle Pathologie und Pharmakologie*, **251**:189–190 (in German).

Rusch GM, Clary JJ, Rinehart WE, Bolte HF (1983) A 26-week inhalation toxicity study with formaldehyde in the monkey, rat, and hamster. *Toxicology and Applied Pharmacology*, **68**:329–343.

Schlosser PM, Lilly PD, Conolly RB, Janszen DB, Kimbell JS (2003) Benchmark dose risk assessment for formaldehyde using airflow modeling and a single-compartment, DNA–protein cross-link dosimetry model to estimate human equivalent doses. *Risk Analysis*, **23**:473–487.

Sewell BT, Bouloukos C, von Holt C (1984) Formaldehyde and glutaraldehyde in the fixation of chromatin for electron microscopy. *Journal of Microscopy*, **136**:103–112.

Shaham J, Bomstein Y, Gurvich R, Rashkovsky M, Kaufman Z (2003) DNA–protein crosslinks and p53 protein expression in relation to occupational exposure to formaldehyde. *Occupational and Environmental Medicine*, **60**:403–409.

Soffritti M, Maltoni C, Maffei F, Biagi R (1989) Formaldehyde: An experimental multipotential carcinogen. *Toxicology and Industrial Health*, **5**:699–730.

Speit G, Schutz P, Merk O (2000) Induction and repair of formaldehyde-induced DNA–protein crosslinks in repair-deficient human cell lines. *Mutagenesis*, **15**:85–90.

St Clair MB, Gross EA, Morgan KT (1990) Pathology and cell proliferation induced by intra-nasal instillation of aldehydes in the rat: Comparison of glutaraldehyde and formaldehyde. *Toxicologic Pathology*, **18**:353–361.

St Clair MB, Bermudez E, Gross EA, Butterworth BE, Recio L (1991) Evaluation of the genotoxic potential of glutaraldehyde. *Environmental and Molecular Mutagenesis*, **18**:113–119.

Stroup NE, Blair A, Erikson GE (1986) Brain cancer and other causes of deaths in anatomists. *Journal of the National Cancer Institute*, **77**:1217–1224.

Swenberg JA, Gross EA, Martin J, Popp JA (1983) Mechanisms of formaldehyde toxicity. In: Gibson JE, ed. *Formaldehyde toxicity*. Washington, DC, Hemisphere Publishing, pp. 132–147.

Swenberg JA, Gross EA, Martin J, Randall HA (1986) Localization and quantitation of cell proliferation following exposure to nasal irritants. In: Barrow CS, ed. *Toxicology of the nasal passages*. Washington, DC, Hemisphere Publishing, pp. 291–300.

Takahashi M, Hasegawa R, Furukawa F, Toyoda K, Sato H, Hayashi Y (1986) Effects of ethanol, potassium metabisulfite, formaldehyde and hydrogen peroxide on gastric carcinogenesis in rats after initiation with *N*-methyl-*N'*-nitro-*N*-nitrosoguanidine. *Japanese Journal of Cancer Research*, **77**:118–124.

Til HP, Woutersen RA, Feron VJ, Hollanders VHM, Falke HE (1989) Two-year drinking-water study of formaldehyde in rats. *Food and Chemical Toxicology*, **27**:77–87.

Titenko-Holland N, Levine AJ, Smith MT, Quintana PJ, Boeniger M, Hayes R, Suruda A, Schulte P (1996) Quantification of epithelial cell micronuclei by fluorescence in situ hybridization (FISH) in mortuary science students exposed to formaldehyde. *Mutation Research*, **371**:237–248.

Tobe M, Naito K, Kurokawa Y (1989) Chronic toxicity study on formaldehyde administered orally to rats. *Toxicology*, **56**:79–86.

Uotila L, Koivusalo M (1974) Formaldehyde dehydrogenase from human liver. Purification, properties, and evidence for the formation of glutathione thiol esters by the enzyme. *Journal of Biological Chemistry*, **249**:7653–7663.

Uotila L, Koivusalo M (1997) Expression of formaldehyde dehydrogenase and *S*-formylglutathione hydrolase activities in different rat tissues. *Advances in Experimental Medicine and Biology*, **414**:365–371.

Van Miller JP, Hermansky SJ, Neptun DA, Loscoa PE, Ballantyne B (1995) Combined chronic toxicity/oncogenicity study with glutaraldehyde (GA) in the drinking water of rats. *Toxicologist*, **15**:203 (abstract).

Vargová M, Janota S, Karelová J, Barancokova M, Šulcová M (1992) Analysis of the health risk of occupational exposure to formaldehyde using biological markers. *Analysis*, **20**:451–454.

Vock EH, Lutz WK, Ilinskaya O, Vamvakas S (1999) Discrimination between genotoxicity and cytotoxicity for the induction of DNA double-strand breaks in cells treated with aldehydes and diepoxides. *Mutation Research*, **441**:85–93.

Walrath J, Fraumeni JF Jr (1983) Mortality patterns among embalmers. *International Journal of Cancer*, **31**:407–411.

Wolf DC, Gross EA, Lycht O, Bermudez E, Recio L, Morgan KT (1995) Immunohistochemical localization of p53, PCNA, and TGF-α proteins in formaldehyde-induced rat nasal squamous cell carcinomas. *Toxicology and Applied Pharmacology*, **132**:27–35.

Woutersen RA, van Garderen-Hoetmer A, Bruijntjes JP, Zwart A, Feron VJ (1989) Nasal tumours in rats after severe injury to the nasal mucosa and prolonged exposure to 10 ppm formaldehyde. *Journal of Applied Toxicology*, **9**:39–46.

Ying C-J, Yan W-S, Zhao M-Y, Ye X-L, Xie H, Yin S-Y, Zhu X-S (1997) Micronuclei in nasal mucosa, oral mucosa and lymphocytes in students exposed to formaldehyde vapor in anatomy class. *Biomedical and Environmental Science*, **10**:451–455.

Zeiger E, Gollapudi B, Spencer P (2005) Genetic toxicity and carcinogenicity studies of glutaraldehyde—A review. *Mutation Research*, **589**:136–151.

Zissu D, Gagnaire F, Bonnet P (1994) Nasal and pulmonary toxicity of glutaraldehyde in mice. *Toxicology Letters*, **71**:53–62.

Zissu D, Bonnet P, Binet S (1998) Histopathological study in B6C3F1 mice chronically exposed by inhalation to glutaraldehyde. *Toxicology Letters*, **95**:131–139.

Zwart A, Woutersen RA, Wilmer JWGM, Spit BJ, Feron VJ (1988) Cytotoxic and adaptive effects in rat nasal epithelium after 3-day and 13-week exposure to low concentrations of formaldehyde vapour. *Toxicology*, **51**:87–99.

Appendix: Summary of studies on micronuclei and chromosomal aberrations in humans exposed to formaldehyde (IARC, 2005).

Reference	Target tissue	End-point	Response (control vs exposed)	Comments and exposures
Vargová et al. (1992)	PBL	CA	3.6% vs 3.08%	*n* = 20; high frequency in controls; wood splinter manufacture; formaldehyde 8-h TWA 0.55–10.36 mg/m³ 5–>16 years
Ballarin et al. (1992)	Nasal mucosa	MN	0.25 ± 0.22% vs 0.90 ± 0.47% (*P* < 0.01)	Concurrent exposure to wood dust; no dose–response
Burgaz et al. (2001)	Nasal mucosa	MN	0.61 ± 0.27% vs 1.01 ± 0.62% (*P* < 0.01)	Exposed, *n* = 23; non-exposed, *n* = 27; no dose–response
Burgaz et al. (2002)	Oral mucosa	MN	0.33 ± 0.30% vs 0.71 ± 0.56% pathology laboratory (*P* < 0.05) 0.33 ± 0.30% vs 0.62 ± 0.45% shoe factory (*P* < 0.05)	Exposed, *n* = 22 variable exposures; *n* = 28 exposed to formaldehyde; non-exposed, *n* = 28; correlation with duration of exposure
Titenko-Holland et al. (1996)	Oral mucosa	MN	0.6 ± 0.5% vs 2.0 ± 2.0% (*P* = 0.007)	Exposed, *n* = 28; pre- versus post-exposure; no details on smoking habits; formaldehyde concentrations:
	Nasal mucosa	MN	2.0 ± 1.3% vs 2.5 ± 1.3% (NS)	Oral: 1.2 mg/m³-h vs 18 mg/m³-h, 90 days Nasal: 2.4 mg/m³-h vs 20 mg/m³-h, 90 days
Ying et al. (1997)	Nasal mucosa	MN	1.20 ± 0.67 vs 3.84 ± 1.48 (*P* < 0.001)	Exposed, *n* = 25; pre- versus post-exposure; questions about controlling for age, sex, and smoking habits; formaldehyde concentrations 0.508 ± 0.299 mg/m³ vs 0.012 ± 0.0025 mg/m³
	Oral mucosa	MN	0.57 ± 0.32 vs 0.86 ± 0.56 (*P* < 0.001)	
	PBL	MN	0.91 ± 0.39 vs 1.11 ± 0.54 (NS)	
He et al. (1988)	PBL	CA	3.40 ± 1.57% vs 5.96 ± 2.40% (*P* < 0.01)	Chromosomal aberrations included breaks and gaps, which renders interpretation difficult
		MN	3.15 ± 1.46% vs 6.38 ± 2.50% (*P* < 0.01)	

CA, chromosomal aberrations; MN, micronuclei; NS, not significant; PBL, peripheral blood lymphocytes; TWA, time-weighted average.

PART 2

IPCS FRAMEWORK FOR ANALYSING THE RELEVANCE OF A NON-CANCER MODE OF ACTION FOR HUMANS

PREFACE

Following completion of the IPCS Framework for Analysing the Relevance of a Cancer Mode of Action for Humans (see Part 1), an expert meeting was convened in Geneva in 2006 to explore the question as to whether the IPCS framework could be applied in chemical risk assessment generally (i.e. to develop a non-cancer framework). The participants at this expert meeting concluded that the framework should be applicable to all end-points and proceeded to author a draft publication out of session. The draft was sent for peer review by the members of the Harmonization Project Steering Committee and subsequently revised by the authors, taking into account the peer review comments received.

LIST OF CONTRIBUTORS

Alan R. Boobis
Section of Experimental Medicine and Toxicology, Division of Medicine, Imperial College London, Hammersmith Campus, London, United Kingdom

John E. Doe
European Centre for Ecotoxicology and Toxicology of Chemicals (ECETOC), Brussels, Belgium

Barbara Heinrich-Hirsch
Safety of Substances and Preparations, Federal Institute for Risk Assessment, Berlin, Germany

M.E. (Bette) Meek
Existing Substances Division, Safe Environments Programme, Health Canada, Ottawa, Ontario, Canada

Sharon Munn
Toxicology and Chemical Substances, Institute for Health and Consumer Protection, Joint Research Centre, European Chemicals Bureau, Ispra, Italy

Mathuros Ruchirawat
Chulabhorn Research Institute (CRI), Lak Si, Bangkok, Thailand

Josef Schlatter
Nutritional and Toxicological Risks Section, Swiss Federal Office of Public Health, Zurich, Switzerland

Jennifer Seed
Risk Assessment Division, Environmental Protection Agency, Washington, DC, USA

Carolyn Vickers
International Programme on Chemical Safety, World Health Organization, Geneva, Switzerland

LIST OF ACRONYMS AND ABBREVIATIONS

ACE	angiotensin-converting enzyme
CSAF	chemical-specific adjustment factor
EMS	eosinophilia-myalgia syndrome
HBOC	haemoglobin-based oxygen carriers
HRF	Human Relevance Framework
ILO	International Labour Organization
ILSI	International Life Sciences Institute
IPCS	International Programme on Chemical Safety
MOA	mode of action
MPTP	1-methyl-4-phenyl-1,2,3,6-tetrahydropyridine
RSI	Risk Science Institute (ILSI)
SLE	systemic lupus erythematosus
UNEP	United Nations Environment Programme
WHO	World Health Organization

IPCS FRAMEWORK FOR ANALYSING THE RELEVANCE OF A NON-CANCER MODE OF ACTION FOR HUMANS[1]

Alan R. Boobis, John E. Doe, Barbara Heinrich-Hirsch, M.E. (Bette) Meek, Sharon Munn, Mathuros Ruchirawat, Josef Schlatter, Jennifer Seed, & Carolyn Vickers

Structured frameworks are extremely useful in promoting transparent, harmonized approaches to the risk assessment of chemicals. One area where this has been particularly successful is in the analysis of modes of action (MOAs) for chemical carcinogens in experimental animals and their relevance to humans. The International Programme on Chemical Safety (IPCS) recently published an updated version of its MOA Framework in animals to address human relevance (cancer Human Relevance Framework, or HRF). This work has now been extended to non-cancer effects, with the eventual objective of harmonizing framework approaches to both cancer and non-cancer end-points. As in the cancer HRF, the first step is to determine whether the weight of evidence based on experimental observations is sufficient to establish a hypothe-sized MOA. This comprises a series of key events causally related to the toxic effect, identi-fied using an approach based on the Bradford Hill criteria. These events are then compared qualitatively and, next, quantitatively between experimental animals and humans. The output of the analysis is a clear statement of conclusions, together with the confidence, analysis, and implications of the findings. This framework provides a means of ensuring a transparent eval-uation of the data, identification of key data gaps and of information that would be of value in the further risk assessment of the compound, such as on dose–response relationships, and recognition of potentially susceptible subgroups, for example, based on life stage considera-tions.

The framework described in this paper, a non-cancer Human Relevance Framework (HRF), was prepared by the International Programme on Chemical Safety (IPCS) (WHO/ILO/UNEP) project on the Harmonization of Approaches to the Assessment of Risk from Exposure to Chemicals. This global "Harmonization Project" aims to harmonize global approaches to chemical risk assessment through both increased consistency of risk assessment methodologies and development of international guidance documents. The project enables the achievement of commitments on harmonization of chemical risk assessment methodologies agreed by the United Nations Conference on Environment and Development (United Nations, 1992), the Intergovernmental Forum on Chemical Safety (1994), the World Summit on Sustainable Development (UNEP, 2002), and the Strategic Approach to International Chemicals Management (WHO, 2006). The project involves experts from the different sectors where chemicals are assessed, and hence the documents produced can be applied in the assessment of industrial chemicals, biocides, pesticides, veterinary chemicals, pharmaceuticals, cosmetics, natural toxicants, food additives, and environmental contaminants in food, water, air, and consumer products.

A main outcome of the Harmonization Project is the IPCS Conceptual Framework for Evaluating a Mode of Action for Chemical Carcinogenesis (Sonich-Mullin et al., 2001) and

---

[1] This article, to which WHO owns copyright, was published in 2008 in *Critical Reviews in Toxicology*, Volume 38, pages 87–96. It has been edited for this WHO publication.

its subsequent development into an IPCS Framework for Analysing the Relevance of a Cancer Mode of Action for Humans (IPCS cancer HRF) (Boobis et al., 2006; see also Part 1 of this document). The mode-of-action (MOA) analysis utilizes a weight-of-evidence approach based on the Bradford Hill criteria for causality (Hill, 1965). It aims to determine whether it is possible to establish an MOA for a carcinogenic response observed in an experimental animal study, through application of a weight-of-evidence approach that requires identification of key events along the causal pathway to cancer. When an MOA has been established in experimental animals, the cancer HRF provides an analytical tool to enable the transparent evaluation of the data in order to consider the human relevance of the MOA.

Following on from this, IPCS decided to consider whether the framework for cancer could be applied, with modifications, if necessary, to other end-points and their associated MOAs. Recognizing the work that the Risk Science Institute (RSI) of the International Life Sciences Institute (ILSI) had conducted in parallel to develop a similar framework and apply it to non-cancer risk assessment, IPCS convened an international meeting in Geneva in March 2006 to review and consider the ILSI publication (Seed et al., 2005), along with the IPCS cancer HRF (Boobis et al., 2006; see also Part 1 of this document), in order to explore the question as to whether the IPCS framework could be applied in chemical risk assessment generally. In summary, this IPCS meeting recognized that the framework should be applicable to all end-points, both cancer and non-cancer, and recommended further work to put this into practice, including documenting the rationale for application of the framework more generally, which appears in the present paper, and steps to facilitate uptake and use of the framework.

The IPCS meeting recognized that the non-cancer HRF would have multiple uses in chemical risk assessment:

- It would provide an internationally harmonized approach to the establishment of an MOA in experimental animals and its relevance to humans.
- It would generate criteria for the MOA against which subsequent cases could be considered—that is, to show whether a compound shares an established MOA.
- It would enable clarification of key information relating to the human relevance of the MOA, and this would inform the assessment of other chemicals that share the MOA.
- In general, application of the framework would enable critical data deficiencies and research needs to be identified and inform qualitative and quantitative assessment.

THE NEED FOR A NON-CANCER HUMAN RELEVANCE FRAMEWORK

The non-cancer HRF is a tool that provides a structured approach to the assessment of human relevance of a postulated MOA in animals in a weight-of-evidence context. Subsequently, it includes explicit consideration of the relevance of the proposed MOA to humans, often based on consideration of more generic information, such as anatomical, physiological, and biochemical variations among species. In this manner, the framework encourages maximum use of both chemical-specific and more generic information in a transparent and analytical fashion.

Pivotal to transparency in determining human relevance using the framework are the delineation and consideration of the nature of evidence in various species of key events—that is, those in a postulated MOA that are measurable and critical to the induction of the toxicological response. Evaluation of the concordance of key events based on explicit consideration of variations between experimental animals and humans constitutes the principal basis of transparency in consideration of weight of evidence for human relevance.

While principally relevant to hazard characterization, the non-cancer HRF additionally contributes more generally to transparency in risk assessment through explicit delineation and consideration of data on appropriate key events that are also relevant to subsequent dose–response analysis for MOAs deemed relevant to humans. If the MOA in experimental animals is judged to be qualitatively relevant to humans, a more quantitative assessment is required that takes into account any kinetic and dynamic information that is available from both the experimental animals and humans in order to determine whether human relevance might be precluded on this basis.

These same data are critical to subsequent dose–response analysis for MOAs considered relevant in considering the adequacy of, for example, available information as a basis for replacement of default uncertainty factors in the development of chemical-specific adjustment factors (CSAFs) (IPCS, 2005). This information could, for example, constitute an adequate basis to consider interspecies variation in rates of formation of reactive metabolites in the target tissue, for replacement of the default subfactor for interspecies differences in toxicokinetics with a CSAF (IPCS, 2005).

Use of this non-cancer HRF also promotes harmonization of approaches to risk assessment for all end-points, bridging previously distinct approaches on, for example, cancer and non-cancer effects. Harmonization in this context refers to a biologically consistent approach to risk assessment for all end-points, for which exploration of biological linkages is critical to ensuring maximal use of relevant information. Often, for example, organ toxicity is a critical key event in postulated MOAs for induction of tumours at the same site. The non-cancer HRF, then, sets the stage for identification of critical precursor non-cancer key events for which subsequent quantification of interspecies differences and interindividual variability in dose–response analysis is relevant. In other cases, a postulated MOA may lead to toxic effects in multiple organs, and these would be considered in the same non-cancer HRF analysis.

In addition, consideration in a transparent framework may identify factors that, while not themselves essential for the toxicological effect (and hence not key events), may modulate key events and, as a result, contribute to differences between species or individuals. Such factors include genetic differences in pathways of metabolism, competing pathways of metabolism, and cell proliferation induced by concurrent pathology.

Such an analysis may also provide an indication of those components of a proposed MOA that may operate only over a certain dose range. If a high experimental dose of a given compound is needed to result in an obligatory step in an MOA, then the relevance to human risk becomes a matter of exposure. Thus, the exposure assessment step of the risk assessment is critical to a comprehensive evaluation.

Importantly, then, application of the non-cancer HRF contributes to identification of any specific subpopulations (e.g. those with genetic predisposition) who are at increased risk and provides information relevant to consideration of relative risks at various life stages. In many cases, this is based not on chemical-specific information but rather on inference, based on knowledge of the MOA, as to whether specific age groups may be at increased or decreased risk. This requires explicit consideration of comparative developmental and ageing processes and events in humans and animal models. These considerations are critical to determination of focus in the remaining stages of risk assessment, such as dose–response analysis.

The transparent delineation of the weight of evidence for postulated MOAs and their relevance to humans (requiring explicit consideration of the strengths and weaknesses of the available database, as well as highlighting qualitative and quantitative similarities and differences among species and related uncertainties) also identifies any inconsistencies in the available data and defines critical data gaps and research needs. This derives from the requirement in each step to explicitly assess confidence in the quality and quantity of data underlying the analysis, consistency of the analysis within the framework, consistency of the database—that is, that studies are not contradictory of each other—and the nature and extent of the concordance analysis.

Iterative application of the non-cancer HRF, even before all of the data are available, to the analysis of a postulated MOA and its relevance to humans are beneficial as a basis for developing and refining research strategies as additional information becomes available. In this context, the framework should prove helpful in facilitating discussion between risk assessors and research scientists in jointly understanding the nature of data that would support human relevance analysis of a postulated MOA in animals and defining next steps in data acquisition. Iterative consideration of MOA in designing research strategies is also expected to increase efficiency by focusing resources in critical areas in more tiered and targeted approaches.

As knowledge advances, MOAs will become less chemical specific and based even more on the key biological processes involved, allowing greater generalization of human relevance from one compound to another. The need for chemical-specific data for established MOAs will be less, although it will always be necessary to establish rigorously that the key events comprising the MOA occur.

The transparency in the human relevance of a postulated MOA that results from application of the non-cancer HRF should promote confidence in the conclusions reached, through the use of a defined procedure that encourages clear and consistent documentation supporting the analysis and reasoning, highlights inconsistencies and uncertainties in the available data, and identifies critically important data gaps that, when filled, would increase confidence in outcome. This transparency not only is anticipated to facilitate discussion between the risk assessment and research communities, but may also contribute to greater convergence among different regulatory agencies.

110

The non-cancer HRF also provides the basis for improved process and content for scientific peer input and peer review, specifying minimum criteria of clarity and transparency as a basis to acquire input and acceptance of postulated MOAs and their relevance to humans. Adherence to these criteria enables others to determine the basis of the conclusions reached with respect to the key events, the exclusion of other MOAs, and the analysis of human relevance.

WHEN WOULD THE NON-CANCER HRF BE APPLIED?

The non-cancer HRF provides a valuable tool to assess an MOA, but it requires significant amounts of effort and experimental work, so it is not something that would be used during the course of the assessment of every chemical. Its main purpose would be to determine whether to apply the default assumption that all effects seen in animals are relevant to humans. This question increases in importance when the application of the default assumption during the course of a risk assessment indicates that adverse effects are likely to occur—for example, where there is a low margin of exposure between the point of departure for the effect under consideration and the estimated human exposure, especially if the human exposure estimate has already been refined. It then becomes important to know whether risk management measures will be required. This is of most concern when new data emerge, such as those identifying a new effect, additional data on the dose–response relationship of the chemical, or changes in use pattern or exposure estimation, which change the risk assessment of a chemical that is already in use.

Use of the non-cancer HRF may also be of value in the situation where the effects in animals would have potentially serious consequences if they occurred in humans, such as neurotoxicity or teratogenesis. These effects are subject to very rigorous risk assessment procedures, so they comparatively frequently suggest the need for risk management measures.

Another situation in which use of the non-cancer HRF should be considered is where there are interspecies differences in either the type of effect or the dose levels at which an effect occurs. In these cases, it will be important to understand which species is the most appropriate upon which to base extrapolation to humans. This indication would also apply to differences between sexes or strains in the same species.

These situations indicate that further consideration is required, and the non-cancer HRF provides a way of doing this. The framework can be applied at any stage in the process of considering an effect. It should be applied in an iterative way during the course of investigating an effect to help guide the scientist. When an effect has first been observed and gives rise to concern, the framework allows the investigator to structure the work programme by prompting the questions to be addressed. As the investigation develops, it guides the investigator in assessing the data as they are generated and provides pointers in deciding whether and what other data would be required.

In situations where there is a large body of data, the framework allows the evaluator to weight the evidence according to its significance as well as its volume.

The non-cancer HRF can also be useful when a chemical is observed to cause an effect suspected of being caused by an MOA that has already been established using the framework or shares structural similarity to a chemical or class of chemicals with an established MOA. The earlier use of the non-cancer HRF to establish this MOA will have identified the key steps that need to be investigated in order to ascribe the MOA to the new chemical. This will prove valuable both in a prospective way in designing new research or testing programmes and retrospectively in evaluating a data set.

CONSIDERATION OF THE NON-CANCER HRF

The non-cancer HRF is an analytical tool that enables a structured approach to the assessment of the overall weight of the evidence for the postulated MOA and its relevance to humans. The framework is not designed to provide an absolute answer on sufficiency of the information, as this will vary, depending on the circumstance. It must be emphasized that it is not a checklist of criteria but an approach to data evaluation and presentation. The output from the application of the framework serves as the basis for the continuation of the risk assessment of the compound.

It is envisaged that the non-cancer HRF will be applicable to a wide range of toxicological end-points, encompassing changes in structure and function of organs, tissues, and cells, including physiological and neurobehavioural effects. The types of toxicity that could be addressed using the framework include, but are not limited to:

- *Organ toxicity*: Examples include benzene-induced haematotoxicity (aplastic anaemia), paraquat-induced lung toxicity, chloroquine-induced ocular toxicity.
- *Reproductive toxicity*: Examples include phthalate-induced male infertility, dioxin-induced dysregulation of female fertility.
- *Developmental toxicity*: Examples include methylmercury-induced developmental neurotoxicity, retinoid-induced teratogenesis.
- *Neurotoxicity*: Examples include lead-induced peripheral neuropathy, acrylamide-induced axonopathy, 1-methyl-4-phenyl-1,2,3,6-tetrahydropyridine (MPTP)-induced Parkinson disease.
- *Immunotoxicity*: Examples include organotin-induced immunosuppression, isoniazid-induced systemic lupus erythematosus (SLE)-like syndrome, contaminated L-tryptophan-induced eosinophilia-myalgia syndrome (EMS).

Introduction to MOA

Prior to embarking on a non-cancer HRF analysis, there needs to be careful evaluation of the weight of evidence for a toxicological response on exposure to a chemical in experimental animals. The nature of the non-cancer HRF is such that only one MOA is analysed at a time; hence, for example, different toxicological effects associated with chemical administration, even if observed in the same animals, will require separate framework analyses to discern the MOA for each effect. Consistent with species- and tissue-specific variation in metabolic activation and detoxication, there may be poor site concordance for some toxicants. This will need to be kept in mind when comparing animal and human data.

112

Postulated mode of action (theory of the case)

This comprises a brief outline of the sequence of events in the MOA postulated to be responsible for the toxicological effect of the test substance. This description leads into the next section, which identifies the events considered "key" (i.e. necessary and measurable) in the MOA.

Key events

The "key events" in the MOA are briefly identified and described. Key events are those events that are critical to the induction of the toxicological response as hypothesized in the postulated MOA and are also measurable. To support an event as key, there needs to be a body of experimental data in which the event is characterized and consistently measured. The types of information that might be relevant include, for example, toxicological response and relevant key events in the same cell type, sites of action logically related to the event(s), specific biochemical events, changes in the expression or activity of enzymes, receptor–ligand interactions, effects on cofactor levels, specific changes in histology, changes in cell proliferation (increased or decreased), perturbations in hormone homeostasis or other signalling pathways (either intracellular or extracellular), second messengers, or ion fluxes, increased degradation of macromolecules, and changes in membrane permeability or integrity.

Concordance of dose–response relationships

The dose–response relationships for each of the key events and for the toxicological response should be characterized and their interrelationships discussed with respect to the Bradford Hill criteria (Hill, 1965). Ideally, it should be possible to correlate the dose dependency of the increases in the magnitude (or frequency) of a key event with increases in the severity (e.g. lesion progression) of other key events occurring later in the process and with the ultimate toxicological response. Comparative tabular presentation of the magnitude of changes in key events and toxicological response is often helpful in examining dose–response concordance.

It is important to consider whether there are fundamental differences in the biological response (i.e. dose transitions) at different parts of the dose–response curve (Slikker et al., 2004). If so, key events relevant to the different parts of the dose–response curve will need to be defined and used in the framework analysis.

Temporal association

The temporal relationships for each of the key events and for the toxicological response should be characterized. Key events should be observable before toxicity is apparent and should be consistent temporally with each other; this is an essential step in deciding whether the data support the postulated MOA. Observations of key events at the same time as the toxicological response (e.g. at the end of a study) do not permit conclusions as to temporal association, but can contribute to the analysis described in the next section.

Strength, consistency, and specificity of association of toxicological response with key events

The weight of evidence linking the key events, any precursor lesions, and the toxicological response should be addressed (see Weed [2005] for a discussion of what is meant by weight of evidence). Stop/recovery studies showing absence or reduction of toxicity when a key event is blocked or reduced are particularly useful tests of the association. Consistent observations in a number of studies, with different experimental designs, increase support for the MOA, since different designs can reduce any unknown bias or confounding. Consistency, which is the repeatability of the key events in the postulated MOA in different studies, is distinct from coherence, however, which addresses the relationship of the postulated MOA with observations more broadly (see next point). Observations that may be of value here include toxicological response and relevant key events in the same cell type, sites of action logically related to event(s), and results from stop/recovery studies.

Biological plausibility and coherence

One should consider whether the MOA is consistent with what is known about the biology of the target process/site in general (biological plausibility) and also in relation to what is known specifically about the overall biological effects of the substance (coherence). For the postulated MOA and its associated key events to be biologically plausible, they need to be consistent with current understanding of biology. However, when using biological plausibility as a criterion against which weight of evidence is assessed, it is important to consider the potential for gaps in our knowledge. Coherence, which addresses the relationship of the postulated MOA with chemical-specific observations more broadly—for example, association of the MOA for the toxicological response with that for other end-points—needs to be distinguished from consistency (addressed in the preceding point). In assessing coherence, information on structural analogues may be of value (i.e. structure–activity analysis). Information from other compounds that share the postulated MOA may also be helpful, such as sex, species, and strain differences in sensitivity and their relationship to key events. Additionally, this section should consider whether the database on the agent is internally consistent in supporting the proposed MOA.

Other modes of action

Alternative MOAs that logically present themselves should be considered. If alternative MOAs are supported, they will need a separate non-cancer HRF analysis. These should be distinguished from additional components of a single MOA, since these would be addressed as part of the MOA under consideration.

Uncertainties, inconsistencies, and data gaps

Uncertainties should be stated fully and explicitly. They should include those related to the biology of the toxicological response and those for the database on the compound being evaluated. Any inconsistencies should be noted and data gaps identified. It should be clearly stated whether the identified data gaps are critical in supporting the postulated MOA.

Assessment of postulated mode of action

There should be a clear statement of the outcome of the analysis, indicating the level of confidence in the postulated MOA—for example, high, moderate, or low. If a novel MOA is being proposed, this should be clearly indicated. However, if the MOA is the same as one previously described, the extent to which the key events fit this MOA needs to be stated explicitly. Any major differences should be noted and their implications for acceptance of the MOA discussed.

Life stage considerations

Since the response of an organism to a chemical exposure may vary through its lifespan, consideration of life stage is important for the MOA analysis of all toxic end-points. This is particularly true for effects that result from developmental exposures, since organ susceptibility may be restricted to critical periods of development, may depend on the ontogeny of key metabolic enzymes, or may depend on the interaction of the developing organism with its mother (see Zoetis & Walls, 2003). In addition, disruption of developmental processes may have downstream consequences.

Consideration of the ageing process is also important, for several reasons. First, developmental exposures can result in toxicities that are not detected until much later in life. In addition, there can be species-specific patterns of ageing for different organ systems. For example, reproductive senescence has a different etiology in rodents and humans and can even differ among different strains of rodents.

Human relevance

If it is possible to establish an MOA in animals for a toxicological effect, the next stage is to evaluate its relevance to humans. The IPCS non-cancer HRF is presented as an approach to answering a series of three (or four) questions, leading to a documented, logical conclusion regarding the human relevance of the MOA underlying the toxicological effect. The application of the guidance results in a narrative with four (or five) sections, which may be incorporated into the hazard characterization of a risk assessment.

1. Is the weight of evidence sufficient to establish a mode of action (MOA) in animals? This question is addressed by performing an MOA analysis as described above, the steps of which are based on the Bradford Hill criteria for causality (Hill, 1965). The weight of evidence for possible alternative MOAs needs to be considered and a conclusion reached on the overall strength of evidence supporting the MOA under consideration. The approach also identifies any critically important data gaps that, when filled, would increase confidence in the proposed MOA. If the postulated MOA has already been described for other chemicals, its human relevance will already have been evaluated. If the proposed MOA is novel, human relevance will need to be assessed de novo.

2. Can human relevance of the MOA be reasonably excluded on the basis of fundamental, qualitative differences in key events between experimental animals and humans? This step involves a qualitative assessment of the relevance of the MOA to humans. Listing the critical key events that occur in the animal MOA and directly evaluating whether or not each of the key events might occur in humans facilitate the evaluation and increase the transparency of the process. Presentation in tabular form, referred to as a concordance table, can be particularly useful. The information in such tables should be relatively brief, as a narrative explanation should always accompany the table. In one column, the effect on humans for each of the key events is evaluated. Another column for the results in a different strain, species, or sex or for a different route of administration that does not result in toxicity can be useful for comparative purposes. Factors may be identified that, while not key themselves, can modulate key events and so contribute to differences between species or individuals. Examples include genetic differences in pathways of metabolism, competing pathways of metabolism, and effects induced by concurrent pathology. Any such factors identified should be noted in a footnote to the concordance table.

The evaluation of the concordance of the key events for the MOA for a given chemical in humans is an evaluation of the MOA in humans, rather than an evaluation of the specific chemical. In general, details of the initial key events are likely to be more chemical specific. Later events will be more generic to the MOA. While information for evaluating the key events in humans can come from in vitro and in vivo studies on the substance itself, basic information on anatomy, physiology, endocrinology, genetic disorders, epidemiology, and any other information that is known regarding the key events in humans can be of value.

In answering this question, a narrative describing the weight of evidence and an evaluation of the level of confidence for the human information should be prepared. Examples of specific types of information that can be useful include:

- where appropriate, background incidences of the effect at the anatomical site and cell type of interest, including age, sex, ethnic differences, and risk factors, including chemicals and other environmental agents;
- knowledge of the nature and function of the target site, including development, structure (gross and microscopic), and control mechanisms at the physiological, cellular, and biochemical levels;
- human and animal disease states that provide insight concerning target organ regulation and responsiveness;
- human and animal responses to the chemical under review or structural analogues following short-, intermediate-, or long-term exposure, including target organs and effects.

Obviously, a substantial amount of information is required to conclude that a given MOA is not relevant to humans. If such a conclusion is strongly supported by the data, exposure to chemicals producing toxicity only by that MOA would not pose a risk to humans, and no additional risk characterization for this end-point is required.

The question of relevance considers all groups and life stages. It is possible that the conditions under which an MOA operates occur primarily in a susceptible subpopulation or life stage—for example, in those with a pre-existing viral infection, hormonal imbalance, or disease state. Any information suggesting qualitative or quantitative differences in susceptibility is highlighted for use in risk characterization.

There are several aspects relating to life stage that should be considered in the non-cancer HRF analysis. First, the analysis should consider the comparative developmental processes and events that occur in humans and the animal model(s) (see Zoetis & Walls, 2003). This comparison will demonstrate the extent to which developmental processes are similar in humans and the animal model(s). In general, development is highly conserved; where this is the case, it would lead to a conclusion that the MOA in animals is also plausible in humans. However, there are some developmental processes that are unique to some species, which may therefore lead to a species-specific MOA that will not be plausible in humans.

Second, the analysis should consider the phase specificity or relative timing of the developmental processes or events in humans and the animal model(s). Critical developmental events may occur at different times during ontogeny. Some developmental events may occur early during the prenatal development of the animal and relatively late in human prenatal development. Other developmental events may occur prenatally in humans and postnatally in the animal, or vice versa. Differences in timing of the developmental events can have an impact on the dose metrics if there are substantial differences in placental versus lactational transfer. Similarly, a comparison of the ontogeny of key metabolic enzymes relative to the key developmental process may reveal substantial differences between humans and the animal model. Such considerations may lead to a conclusion that the animal MOA is not plausible in humans.

3. Can human relevance of the MOA be reasonably excluded on the basis of quantitative differences in either kinetic or dynamic factors between experimental animals and humans? If the MOA in experimental animals cannot be judged to be qualitatively irrelevant to humans (*no* to question 2), a more quantitative assessment is undertaken, taking into account any kinetic and dynamic information that is available from experimental animals and humans. Such data will of necessity be both chemical and MOA specific and where possible should include the biologically effective doses required to produce the dynamic effects giving rise to the toxicity. Kinetic considerations include the rate and extent of absorption, tissue distribution, metabolism, and excretion. Differences in ontogeny can result in substantial species differences in placental and lactational transfers, which will affect the dose metrics. This may therefore result in a quantitative difference in the MOA between humans and experimental animals. Similarly, the differential ontogeny of key metabolic enzymes can result in substantial quantitative differences between humans and experimental animals. Dynamic considerations include the consequences of the interaction of the chemical with cells, tissues, and organs. Only infrequently is it likely that it will be possible to dismiss human relevance on the basis of quantitative differences. Since quantitative exposure assessment is part of the subsequent risk characterization rather than the HRF, the difference would have to be of such a magnitude that human exposure could not possibly be envisaged to reach such levels. In most cases, it will not be possible to reach such a conclusion without undertaking formal exposure assessment in the subsequent risk characterization. Hence, the answer to the question will be *no*, but it may still be concluded that the risk is negligible in the subsequent risk characterization. Melamine-induced urinary bladder carcinogenesis provides a useful case-study illustrating this point (Meek et al., 2003). Again, tabular comparison of the data from experimental animals and humans can help in the evaluation. Information from studies of other compounds acting by the same or a similar MOA can be of value. As understanding of the basis for differences in responses between experimental animals and humans improves, differences in key events thought to be qualitative may be shown to be due to specific quantitative differences.

While it may not be possible to conclude that the MOA for toxicity is not relevant to humans on the basis of quantitative differences, during the evaluation it may become apparent that the magnitude of those differences is sufficient to impact markedly on the risk assessment. Hence, it is particularly important that the narrative for the answer to this question be comprehensive and capture as much quantitative information as possible.

117

As with question 2, if the response to this question is *yes*, then exposure to chemicals producing toxicity only by this MOA would not pose a risk to humans, and no additional risk characterization is required.

The preceding three questions comprise a decision tree (see Figure 1).

		Is the weight of evidence sufficient to establish a mode of action (MOA) in animals?	**NO** →	Continue with risk assessment

↓ **YES**

MOA not relevant	**YES** ←	Can human relevance of the MOA be reasonably excluded on the basis of fundamental, qualitative differences in key events between experimental animals and humans?		

↓ **NO**

MOA not relevant	**YES** ←	Can human relevance of the MOA be reasonably excluded on the basis of quantitative differences in either kinetic or dynamic factors between experimental animals and humans?	**NO** →	Continue with risk assessment

Figure 1. Decision tree for determining human relevance of an MOA for toxicity observed in experimental animals.

Potential implications for dose–response assessment

Should it not be possible to exclude human relevance of the MOA for toxicity prior to proceeding with the risk assessment, a further question should be addressed. This is: *4. Are there any quantitative differences in the key events such that default values for uncertainty factors for species or individual differences could be modified?* Such information, on either kinetics or dynamics, could be used to calculate a CSAF, in which one or more of the default values for species or interindividual differences in kinetics or dynamics are replaced by a value based on chemical-specific information (IPCS, 2005). The other components of the adjustment factor would retain their default values. Such information may lead to either an increase or a decrease in the adjustment factor relative to the normal default.

Published case-studies

In developing a framework for assessing the human relevance of MOAs for non-cancer endpoints, ILSI/RSI also developed a series of illustrative case-studies. These were on molinate-induced inhibition of spermatogenesis (Kavlock & Cummings, 2005a), renal and developmental effects of ethylene glycol (Corley et al., 2005), developmental neurotoxicity of nicotine (Slikker et al., 2005), phthalate ester effects on male reproductive development (Foster, 2005), vinclozolin-induced malformations (Kavlock & Cummings, 2005b), developmental effects of valproic acid (Wiltse, 2005), haemoglobin-based oxygen carriers (HBOC)-related congenital malformations (Holson et al., 2005), developmental effects of angiotensin-converting enzyme (ACE) inhibitors (Tabacova, 2005), developmental ototoxicity of polyhalogenated aromatic hydrocarbons (Crofton & Zoeller, 2005), and propylthiouracil-induced effects on neurological development (Zoeller & Crofton, 2005). While these cases covered a range of end-points, most involved effects during development. Hence, there is a need for additional case-studies on other end-points, such as those indicated above. As experience is obtained in using this framework, some of the published cases could be further refined to provide valuable illustrative examples for training in the application of the framework.

In general, the cases have been very useful in highlighting a number of the key issues on which this non-cancer HRF is based. Examples include the importance of the concordance analysis, the value of quantitative information identified during the application of the framework when it is not possible to exclude human relevance, the need for a transparent and comprehensive narrative when reporting the conclusions of a framework analysis, the importance in identifying key data gaps (e.g. case-study on molinate and HBOC), identification of research needs (e.g. case-study on vinclozolin), the importance of understanding the formation of a specific metabolite, and the importance of establishing a robust MOA through the application of the Bradford Hill criteria (Hill, 1965) to the key events.

Statement of confidence, analysis, and implications

Following application of the non-cancer HRF and answering the three (or four) questions, a statement of confidence should be provided that addresses the quality and quantity of data underlying the analysis, the consistency of the analysis within the framework, the consistency of the database, and the nature and extent of the concordance analysis. Alternative MOAs should have been evaluated, when appropriate, with the same rigor. A critical outcome is the identification of specific data gaps that could be addressed experimentally to increase confidence in the analysis.

The output of the non-cancer HRF provides information that is useful for more than just determining whether or not the MOA for toxicity in experimental animals is relevant to humans. It can also provide much information that is critically important in subsequent steps in the risk characterization for relevant effects. For example, it may be possible to develop CSAFs on the basis of the information provided. Application of the framework can also provide information on relevant modulating factors that are likely to affect risk. In addition, it can identify those elements of a proposed MOA that operate only over a certain dose range. Where an obligatory step in an MOA occurs only following a high experimental dose of a compound, the relevance of the MOA to human risk is determined by the exposure. Thus, effective exposure assessment is particularly important to the evaluation of human risk from such toxicity.

The analysis also contributes to the identification of any specific subpopulations (e.g. those with genetic predisposition) who may be at increased risk and often provides information useful in considering relative risk at various life stages. This may be based not always on chemical-specific information but rather on inference, on the basis of knowledge of the MOA, as to whether the risk in specific age groups might be expected to differ.

The data and their analysis using the non-cancer HRF should be reported in a clear and comprehensive manner, so that others can determine the basis of the conclusions reached.

Although the specific form of presentation will vary with the type of data available, a structured report, including the key headings from the framework, should be provided where possible. Presentation should include sufficient details on the context and thought processes to ensure transparency of the conclusions reached. The inclusion of concordance tables is strongly encouraged. This increases transparency and facilitates peer engagement.

USE OF THE FRAMEWORK AND ITS OUTPUTS

The IPCS non-cancer HRF, which is based principally on robust concordance analysis of key events in postulated MOAs, is envisaged to be of value to both the risk assessment and research communities as a basis to contribute to harmonization in several areas, including:

- adequacy and nature of weight of evidence for postulated MOAs in animals and their relevance to humans;
- MOA integration across end-points;
- criteria for transparency to ensure sufficiency of peer input and review.

Among the strengths of the non-cancer HRF are its flexibility, transparency, and general applicability across end-points. This includes determination of the nature and shape of the dose–response curve, the identification and location of biological thresholds for individual key events, and their consequences. In addition, consideration of the kinetic and dynamic factors involved in each key event is informative regarding the relevance or not to specific subpopulations—for example, in early life, in those with particular diseases, or in those with specific polymorphisms. Alternatively, application of the framework can provide quantitative information on the differences between such groups. Human relevance analysis may also indicate that a species is inappropriate for evaluating a potentially relevant end-point because of dose limitations.

NEXT STEPS

To ensure effective adoption of the non-cancer HRF, there will be a need to train individuals in its application and in the interpretation of its outputs. Experience is being gained in the use of the cancer HRF, and the expertise gained would be applicable in the training of others in the use of the non-cancer HRF. Training would be facilitated by the availability of a number of suitable case-studies. Those published to date would be a sound basis for further development for this purpose (Seed et al., 2005). In addition, cases on a wider range of end-points need to be developed. It would be helpful if organizations with experience in non-cancer HRF analysis could develop courses and make the materials available to others with suitable expertise to help in training.

A database of generally accepted MOAs should be compiled and maintained, together with informative case-studies. Such a database would be of particular importance as experience continues to evolve in the development of MOAs and in determining whether the MOA for a compound is novel or has been described previously for other compounds.

120

The current non-cancer HRF, which arose out of the IPCS cancer HRF, is focused on non-cancer end-points. However, there are marked similarities in the philosophy and strategy to evaluating cancer and non-cancer effects. It is strongly recommended that one of the next steps in harmonization of risk assessment of chemicals should be the preparation of a unified HRF that is applicable to all toxicological end-points, including cancer. The integration of framework approaches into the risk assessment process should be further elaborated, in which illustrative examples would be of value. Some guidance on problem formulation before embarking on an HRF analysis should be included in such a framework document, as should guidance on the use of the outputs of HRF analysis in risk assessment. For example, during application of the framework, a much deeper understanding of dose–response relationships is often developed, which should be taken forward into hazard characterization. As indicated above, knowledge of any dose transitions is invaluable in interpreting exposure data. Identification of key events in the MOA can provide insight into the sources and magnitude of interspecies and interindividual differences.

REFERENCES

Boobis AR, Cohen SM, Dellarco V, McGregor D, Meek ME, Vickers C, Willcocks D, Farland W (2006) IPCS framework for analyzing the relevance of a cancer mode of action for humans. *Critical Reviews in Toxicology*, **36**:781–792.

Corley RA, Meek ME, Carney EW (2005) Mode of action: Oxalate crystal-induced renal tubule degeneration and glycolic acid-induced dysmorphogenesis—Renal and developmental effects of ethylene glycol. *Critical Reviews in Toxicology*, **35**:691–702.

Crofton KM, Zoeller RT (2005) Mode of action: Neurotoxicity induced by thyroid hormone disruption during development—Hearing loss resulting from exposure to PHAHs. *Critical Reviews in Toxicology*, **35**:757–769.

Foster PM (2005) Mode of action: Impaired fetal Leydig cell function—Effects on male reproductive development produced by certain phthalate esters. *Critical Reviews in Toxicology*, **35**:713–719.

Hill AB (1965) The environment and disease: Association or causation? *Proceedings of the Royal Society of Medicine*, **58**:295–300.

Holson JF, Stump DG, Pearce LB, Watson RE, DeSesso JM (2005) Mode of action: Yolk sac poisoning and impeded histiotrophic nutrition—HBOC-related congenital malformations. *Critical Reviews in Toxicology*, **35**:739–745.

Intergovernmental Forum on Chemical Safety (1994) *The International Conference on Chemical Safety—Final report*. Geneva, World Health Organization (http://www.who.int/ifcs/documents/forums/forum1/en/FI-report_en.pdf).

IPCS (2005) *Chemical-specific adjustment factors for interspecies differences and human variability: Guidance document for use of data in dose/concentration–response assessment*.

Geneva, World Health Organization, International Programme on Chemical Safety (Harmonization Project Document No. 2; http://whqlibdoc.who.int/publications/2005/9241546786_eng.pdf).

Kavlock R, Cummings A (2005a) Mode of action: Reduction of testosterone availability—Molinate-induced inhibition of spermatogenesis. *Critical Reviews in Toxicology*, **35**:685–690.

Kavlock R, Cummings A (2005b) Mode of action: Inhibition of androgen receptor function—Vinclozolin-induced malformations in reproductive development. *Critical Reviews in Toxicology*, **35**:721–726.

Meek ME, Bucher JR, Cohen SM, Dellarco V, Hill RN, Lehman-McKeeman LD, Longfellow DG, Pastoor T, Seed J, Patton DE (2003) A framework for human relevance analysis of information on carcinogenic modes of action. *Critical Reviews in Toxicology*, **33**:591–653.

Seed J, Carney E, Corley R, Crofton K, DeSesso J, Foster P, Kavlock R, Kimmel G, Klaunig J, Meek E, Preston J, Slikker W, Tabacova S, Williams G (2005) Overview: Using mode of action and life stage information to evaluate the human relevance of animal toxicity data. *Critical Reviews in Toxicology*, **35**:663–672.

Slikker W Jr, Andersen ME, Bogdanffy MS, Bus JS, Cohen SD, Conolly RB, David RM, Doerrer NG, Dorman DC, Gaylor DW, Hattis D, Rogers JM, Setzer RW, Swenberg JA, Wallace K (2004) Dose-dependent transitions in mechanisms of toxicity. *Toxicology and Applied Pharmacology*, **201**:203–225.

Slikker W Jr, Xu ZA, Levin ED, Slotkin TA (2005) Mode of action: Disruption of brain cell replication, second messenger, and neurotransmitter systems during development leading to cognitive dysfunction—Developmental neurotoxicity of nicotine. *Critical Reviews in Toxicology*, **35**:703–711.

Sonich-Mullin C, Fielder R, Wiltse J, Baetcke K, Dempsey J, Fenner-Crisp P, Grant D, Hartley M, Knaap A, Kroese D, Mangelsdorf I, Meek E, Rice J, Younes M (2001) IPCS conceptual framework for evaluating a mode of action for chemical carcinogenesis. *Regulatory Toxicology and Pharmacology*, **34**:146–152.

Tabacova S (2005) Mode of action: Angiotensin-converting enzyme inhibition—Developmental effects associated with exposure to ACE inhibitors. *Critical Reviews in Toxicology*, **35**:747–755.

UNEP (2002) *Plan of implementation of the World Summit on Sustainable Development.* New York, NY, United Nations Environment Programme (http://www.un.org/esa/sustdev/documents/WSSD_POI_PD/English/WSSD_PlanImpl.pdf).

United Nations (1992) *Agenda 21: United Nations Conference on Environment and Development.* New York, NY, United Nations Division for Sustainable Development (http://www.un.org/esa/sustdev/documents/agenda21/english/Agenda21.pdf).

Weed DL (2005) Weight of evidence: A review of concept and methods. *Risk Analysis*, **25**:1545–1557.

WHO (2006) *Strategic Approach to International Chemicals Management (SAICM).* Geneva, World Health Organization (http://www.who.int/ipcs/features/iccm_crp.pdf).

Wiltse J (2005) Mode of action: Inhibition of histone deacetylase, altering WNT-dependent gene expression, and regulation of beta-catenin—Developmental effects of valproic acid. *Critical Reviews in Toxicology*, **35**:727–738.

Zoeller RT, Crofton KM (2005) Mode of action: Developmental thyroid hormone insufficiency—Neurological abnormalities resulting from exposure to propylthiouracil. *Critical Reviews in Toxicology*, **35**:771–781.

Zoetis T, Walls I, eds (2003) *Principles and practices for direct dosing of preweaning mammals in toxicity testing and research. A report of the ILSI Risk Science Institute Expert Working Group on Direct Dosing of Preweaning Mammals in Toxicity Testing.* Washington, DC, ILSI Press.

THE HARMONIZATION PROJECT DOCUMENT SERIES

IPCS risk assessment terminology (No. 1, 2004)

Chemical-specific adjustment factors for interspecies differences and human variability: Guidance document for use of data in dose/concentration–response assessment (No. 2, 2005)

Principles of characterizing and applying human exposure models (No. 3, 2005)

Part 1. IPCS framework for analysing the relevance of a cancer mode of action for humans and case-studies; Part 2. IPCS framework for analysing the relevance of a non-cancer mode of action for humans (No. 4, 2007)

To order further copies of monographs in this series, please contact WHO Press,
World Health Organization, 1211 Geneva 27, Switzerland
(Fax No.: +41 22 791 4857; E-mail: bookorders@who.int).
The Harmonization Project Documents are also available on the web at http://www.who.int/ipcs/en/.